The
Weight
Loss
Habit

THE WEIGHT LOSS HABIT

Take Charge of Your Weight

Dr. Tushar Agarwal, M.D.

DISCLAIMER

This book is for informational purposes only, based on the personal experiences of the author. The author does not proclaim that the information contained in this book is universally true and the information given may or may not work for you. You should review the information carefully with your professional health care provider before starting any diet and/or exercise program. You are strongly advised to consult your physician prior to using the information contained in this book if you are pregnant, nursing, taking medication, or have a medical condition. The information in this book is not intended to, diagnose, treat, cure, or prevent any disease. The author expressly disclaims responsibility, and shall have no liability, for any damages, loss, injury, or liability whatsoever, whether direct or indirect, suffered as a result of your reliance on the information contained in this book. All product(s) and company names referred to in this book are trademarks™ or registered® trademarks of their respective holders, and reference to them in this book does not imply any affiliation or association with the author, or endorsement by them.

For Mummy and Papa

Table of Contents

Introduction

"Motivation is what gets you started. Habit is what keeps you going."
—Jim Rohn, American entrepreneur, author and motivational speaker

If you do a Google search for "weight loss," you will get 1,540,000,000 hits. Amazon.com has 263,000 product matches corresponding to the search term "weight loss." Clearly, there is neither a paucity of information nor a dearth of products, related to weight loss. Yet, two thirds of adult Americans are either overweight or obese.

If you look at the broader picture, according to the World Health Organization, 39% of adults worldwide are overweight as of 2014.

It is not as if people are not aware of the problem or that they are not trying to resolve it. At any given point in time, 38% of women and 24% of men in America are attempting to lose weight.

So why are they failing?

Part of the answer lies in habits. Both the source and the solution to obesity can be traced to habits. None of the currently available methods of weight loss addresses this aspect of the problem.

People are not born fat. Nor do they become fat overnight. It is a lifetime of poor habits that causes weight gain. Most people are already aware that if you eat less or exercise more, you will lose weight. It is common sense. Yet, the obesity epidemic keeps on growing.

The usual approaches for weight loss provide specific instructions on diet and exercise. It can work, and does work in most cases. The problem is that these methods stop working as soon as you stop following them. And sooner or later you will stop. How long do you think you can continue to eat low-carb or low-fat diets or do spinning or cycling? At some point, you give up and fall back into the comfortable groove of your old habits. When that happens, the weight loss cycle goes into reverse gear and all the weight you so painstakingly lost is regained. In most cases, you end up weighing more than what you weighed with in the first place. Does this sound familiar? It is the story of millions of people who are trying to lose weight.

How do you get out of this vicious trap?

Habits have the necessary power and resilience to do this job for you. They can take you out of the loss-gain-loss cycle.

The Weight Loss Habit, a collection of individual habits that have been scientifically proven to be responsible for long-term maintenance of weight loss, can help.

In this book, I take you through a step-by-step process that will teach you this method. This in turn will make you lose weight, and even more importantly, help you to maintain the weight loss for life.

My Own Realisation

In 2005 I was oblivious to the issue of obesity, mostly because I had never thought of myself as fat.

One morning, I was waiting for the elevator in the university hospital where I work as a physician. Soon enough, the elevator doors opened and my colleagues started to stream inside. I was probably one of the last ones to enter. The doors closed but the elevator would not go up. Instead, there was a harsh beeping sound from the console of the elevator. Instinctively, everyone turned towards the source of the sound. There was a red flashing sign on the console that said "Weight Exceeded."

It was a piquant situation. Every person in the elevator began to look at one another. With everyone wanting to rush to their offices, no one wanted to budge from their positions. Yet every person in that elevator knew that the only way to get it going was if someone sacrificed his or herself for the cause. A cruel judgment game started. Each person started looking around, trying to identify the weakest link, or in this case, the fattest person in the group. I did the same and noticed that there were at least three or four people whom I would consider really fat. Surely one of these guys could step off, I thought. Then my gaze fell upon my own image in the mirror of the elevator. To my great horror, I realized that I was larger than the persons whom I had just judged.

It was a profound revelation, as I had never considered myself to be fat. In my own eyes, I might have been slightly overweight, but was I fat? No! I noticed that by this time, my fellow elevator riders had also figured out that I was the fattest person on there, as everyone's gaze had settled upon me. Before things could become any more embarrassing, one person pressed the open button on the console and very graciously stepped out of the elevator. The doors closed, the beeping noise and the flashing sign ceased and the elevator was on its way up. Everyone removed their gaze away from me.

However my own eyes remained fixed upon my image in the mirror.

I could not believe how fat I was.

It was only when I had compared myself to the people around me that I realized the enormity of my own body.

The ensuing elevator ride was the longest one of my life.

I knew then that I could not allow this situation to continue any longer. I had to do something about my weight, very soon.

To some, this anecdote may sound insignificant or even a little shallow. But it was a big trigger in my life. One that led to a series of events, culminating in the book that is in your hands right now.

It set me upon a path to lose weight. Over the course of the next two years, I managed to lose 20% of my body weight. And even more importantly, I have successfully maintained that weight loss for more than eight years.

Truth That I Stumbled Upon

Once I made up mind to lose weight, I gathered all the information I could get on the subject. I scoured the internet for information and read medical literature on the subject.

Like most people, my first instinct was to look for an easy and fast way to shed weight. Fortunately, it became obvious very early on that there was no shortcut to weight loss.

An unrelated observation dispelled any hopes that I harbored about a magic bullet for shedding weight.

I noticed that there were many people who were very rich,

even billionaires, and yet they were overweight. This innocuous observation was an eye opener for me. I inferred that if a billionaire could be fat, there was no magic bullet for weight loss. Contrary to the popular saying, I believe money *can* actually buy most things. If some billionaires were still fat, despite their riches, it was a message to me that weight loss wasn't something that could be bought off the shelf.

At the same time, there were enough examples that people all around the world were managing to lose weight. If you search for "Before and After Weight Loss" on Google, you will come across heaps of such people.

These observations made a few things very clear to me.

Weight loss could not be bought, it had to be earned. And it could be earned.

The next logical question was, "How do I manage to do it?"

How To Use This Book

Truth be told, I stumbled my way through weight loss. Far from being smooth, it was a journey filled with ups and downs. After many trials and errors, I managed to lose almost 20% of my body weight and have successfully kept it off for the last eight years.

Over this time I have been badgered by my family and friends to share my weight loss "secret" with them. When I did try to teach them, I became aware that doing something yourself is one thing; teaching someone to do something is an altogether different ball game. It was quite similar to the observation that being a good player and being a good coach are not necessarily the same thing.

I decided that if I were to teach my weight loss methods to

others, I had to be sure that they had scientific validity. You can experiment with anything on yourself but if you are going to advise others to do the same, you'd better be sure. To get the scientific validity for my methods, I started reading medical literature on the subject.

As I went through scientific research on the subject of weight loss, I came across the existence of the National Weight Control Registry (NWCR). It is an online registry that tracks people living in the United States who have lost a large amount of weight and have managed to keep it off for a long time. In effect, this is group of people who have achieved exactly what I had managed to achieve myself: significant, long lasting weight reduction. When I read about the characteristics of the people in this group, I was astonished to find they were doing almost the same things I had been doing for my own weight loss.

As I delved deeper into high-quality medical literature on this subject, I came to the conclusion that the reason for the similarity in my actions and those of the participants of the NWCR was no coincidence. There is only one approach to long-term weight loss. And sooner or later, everyone who manages to do so converges upon this path. The only challenge is to learn how to adopt these behaviors.

I recommend that you read this book cover to cover before implementing the changes yourself. Once you get a complete overview of the program, then you should start following the suggestions given here. After you begin following the instructions, you should come back and revisit the relevant chapters. You will find that reading them again after you have started out will give you new insight in to those recommendations.

CHAPTER ONE

How Did You End Up Here?

"Know from whence you came. If you know whence you came, there are absolutely no limitations to where you can go."
—James Baldwin, American novelist and social critic

You were not born overweight. Yet, today, you are overweight. How did you end up in this situation? It is imperative that you understand the process by which you gained a large amount of excess weight. This is because if you want to shed this excess weight, you have to, by necessity, take the same route in reverse.

There is an inevitability about the process that you have to undergo in order to lose weight. Once you recognize this, you will feel much more at peace and will find it easier to focus on the job ahead.

Calorie Weight Relationship

I will begin by giving you a crash course in food science. I am reminded here of something that Hal Elrod, author of the book *Miracle Morning* has mentioned. He says, the most dangerous words in the English language are, "I know this thing." So, please don't say it yourself, and read the following very carefully!

A calorie, a word that you would have heard and used your-self very often, is a unit of energy. It is equivalent to 4.184 absolute Joules. It is sufficient to remember that calorie denotes energy, whether it is being produced or spent.

The food that we eat is processed by our body to extract the energy present in those foods. The energy itself is contained in three constituents that make up any food source: carbohy-drates (think starch), proteins (think egg whites) and fats (think butter).

These constituents each have a different capability to store energy. In other words, these three provide different amounts of energy per gram of intake.

Protein and carbohydrates each have 4 calories in every gram. However, each gram of fat holds about 9 calories. This is where the story of caloric imbalance starts.

Almost whatever we eat is composed of a combination of the three food classes mentioned above. It is their relative propor-tions that vary. The interplay of the three constituents and their individual share in different foods determines a major part of weight gain and consequently weight loss as well.

Where Do The Calories Go?

The calories produced from food metabolism in the body are spent in three ways. The major component goes into maintain-ing the body. This is called the Resting Energy Expenditure (REE). It accounts for almost 60% of the caloric intake in a person. REE is measured when the person is 100% at rest. Any calories burnt as a result of the slightest of body movements, do not go into the REE account. The key here is that 60% of your caloric intake is spent in background caloric expenditure, one on which you have no control.

REE depends on the size of a person. Larger sized people have an advantage here. The body spends more calories to maintain a larger sized body. Think of your body as a vehicle. The larger the vehicle, greater is the fuel consumption. This is probably the last time in this book that the larger size of a person is advantageous in some manner. From now on, things are going to go downhill for the larger sized people!

The second component of caloric expenditure is the thermic effect of food (TEF). It refers to the calories spent by the body in trying to process the foods themselves to produce energy. It accounts for digestion, absorption and storage of energy. This part takes up another 10% of the caloric intake. Think of the energy bill of a power plant. A power plant produces electricity, but to do so, it uses up certain amount of electricity itself. Thermic effect of food is similar. It is the energy spent by the body in producing energy.

At this point, 70% of the caloric expenditure has been accounted for, and still there is no sign of your active contribution. The third component of energy expenditure will fill that gap. It belongs to the broad heading of physical activity. Don't confuse it with exercise. They are different. Exercise is a subset of physical exercise. This is an important distinction and requires further explanation. I will leave it at this for the moment and shall come back to the differentiation between the two later in the book.

For the moment, it will suffice to remember that the broad heading of physical activity accounts for 30% of your caloric expenditure. It is this segment that is almost fully under your control. So, during the course of this book, energy expenditure through physical activity will remain a primary focus.

Weight Equation

"The simplest things are often the truest."

—Richard Bach, American writer

1 Pound = 3500 Calories

Keeping aside the finer nuances, it is a fact that one pound of body weight equals 3,500 calories. If you consume an extra 3,500 calories, you will gain one pound of body weight. In the same vein, if you want to lose one pound of weight, just reverse the equation. Somehow create a caloric loss of 3,500 calories and you will lose one pound of body weight. It really is that simple.

It is a straightforward equation and a simple truth, and yet people try all their might to circumvent it. You can see it in the form of books and weight loss programs that claim that you can lose weight and yet eat whatever and how much you can while doing so. To put it plainly, it is lie. If you are looking to shed weight, there is no going around the weight loss equation. You won't have to starve, but you will need to eat intelligently.

I was lucky in that I understood the true meaning and implication of this equation right at the beginning of my own weight loss journey. It is my belief that my understanding of this concept was the foundation on which my entire success was based.

Your body works like a bank account. Every single calorie that you consume goes on the credit side of the account. Similarly, every calorie that you burn goes on the debit side. Every time the positive balance hits 3,500 calories, you put on one pound of weight. On the opposite side, when the net deficit reaches 3,500 calories, you lose one pound of weight. It is really this simple.

This is a simplified explanation of the calorie-weight equation. I should clarify here that if one were to go into minute detail, this equation has some aberrations. I will touch upon those at a later point in the book. But for most part, this equation works well for most people, most of the time.

The practical use of this equation will come up repeatedly in this book. Every time you look at a food item, your mind should apply this equation. Similarly, every opportunity to burn off calories should bring up this equation. Whenever you see any reference to weight, both in loss or gain terms, you should apply this equation to test the veracity of that claim.

Understanding the Implications of the Weight Loss Equation

Imagine that you're driving a car and you suddenly notice that there is a strange noise coming from the engine. You have never heard this sound before. Anyone who drives a car knows that a new noise from the engine usually means trouble. If you're like most people, your initial reaction is to try and wish it away. "Maybe something is stuck to the tire," you might think. Or, a pebble might have gotten under the hood." You think of any number of ways to explain the noise with a simple, self-limiting explanation. You might even stop the car and restart it in the hope that the noise will go away. If you are one of the hands-on type, you stop the car, open the hood and try to figure out the source of the noise. In short, you try everything that might save you the impending trip to the auto shop.

Rarely, one of these tricks might work to eliminate the noise. Maybe, there was something stuck to the tire after all! But chances of the noise going away on its own are really slim.

On most occasions, you would end up taking the car to the auto shop to get it checked out by a professional. Let's continue to extend this hypothetical situation. The mechanic takes one look at the engine, points out to a broken cable and tells you that it needs to be replaced. He then gives you a price estimate of $300.

At this point, for, you feel the hit, if only for a moment. But something else also happens. A calm descends upon you. You are at peace now. The source of the problem has been identified and the solution to the problem is in front of you. It may cost time and money, but at least you have peace of mind.

You stop trying tricks, which now appear silly, to get the car working.

How is this scenario relevant to weight loss?

Similarly, now that you have noticed the noise (excess weight), you can try and avoid getting the new cable (weight loss equation), but in the end, you will have to come around to doing it. This is why it is so important to fully understand the significance of this equation. Because until you do so, your mind will keep looking for easy tricks and shortcuts to reduce your weight. Anything that might help you avoid changing that cable.

Most people I know like a shortcut. The path of least resistance is the easiest to follow. But once you understand the weight loss equation, you will immediately start to see things in a new light. Claims like, "lose 10 pounds in two weeks" or "eat your way to weight loss" will immediately fall flat in front of you. Your mind will stop wandering to shortcuts.

Why Do We Gain Weight

Before you can begin to lose weight, it is helpful to understand how you gained weight in the first place. Once you understand that weight gain itself is no overnight process, but is a straightforward physical equation, you will be convinced that in order to lose weight, you simply need to reverse your habits.

An average person needs to consume about 2,000 calories per day to sustain his body at any given level of weight. At that level of consumption and with average daily activity, one neither gains nor loses weight.

In most people the level of calorie consumption is a little more than what their bodies burn everyday. So, even an extra 20 calories per day (just 1% of the daily consumption) leads to an excess of 600 calories a month or 7,000 calories per year, assuming that the level of physical activity remains the same during that period. This equates to a gain of around two pounds every year. If this process were to continue unabated for many years, you can see where it would lead.

James Hill, one of the founders of the NWCR, wrote a seminal paper in the journal *Science* where he estimated that the root cause of the American obesity epidemic can be traced to a daily caloric accumulation of 50 calories per person. That is right — the obesity epidemic that America has been struggling with for so many years can be traced to an imbalance of only 50 calories a day. The consequences of this epidemic are not very obvious as they are happening silently. A 2014 report by McKinsey Global

Institute estimated that the obesity epidemic is the costing the United States 117 billion dollars every year. Almost 1 in 5 deaths in America since 1986 is now attributable to obesity. And the cause for all this damage is an imbalance of a mere 50 calories.

Coming back to the individual level, it is evident that you can gain a substantial amount of weight provided you just give it time. It is a very slow, creeping process.

Most people gain weight over a long period of time. Yet, almost all of them, including you, want to shed it very quickly. You want to get rid of it much faster than you accumulated it in the first place. Well, one thing is certain: it will not happen that way.

Weight is gained one calorie at a time and will be shed off one calorie at a time too.

Don't be disheartened by these facts. It is not all gloomy; there is a silver lining. It is true that you may not lose the excess weight overnight, but don't despair that you require the same amount of time to lose the weight as you took to gain it. It may take some time, but it will be much less than the time you spent in gaining it. This is because while you put on excess weight passively you will lose weight proactively.

Proaction trumps passivity every single time.

Why Does Weight Gain Go Unnoticed

We are used to seeing ourselves in the mirror every day. Over a period of time, a particular body image of ourselves gets burned into our consciousness. And since we are looking at ourselves every day, we fail to notice the subtle, incremental changes occurring in our bodies.

In 2006, Pew Research Center, a nonpartisan fact tank, asked a representative nationwide sample of adult Americans what they felt about the weight problem in America. In the survey, nine-in-ten respondents said that most of their fellow Americans were overweight. The number dropped to seven-in-ten, when they were asked about the epidemic amongst "the people they know." And when the question came to their perception of their own weight, people were most forgiving. Less than four-in-ten (39%) said that they themselves were overweight. When you compare this number with the actual figures in America (6 out of 10 Americans are overweight), you realize that almost 30% of overweight people don't even realize it.

People around us, our families, friends and coworkers, get accustomed to seeing us every day. Since weight gain is a very gradual process and we put on only a few grams a day, there isn't a drastic change in our appearance overnight. Consequently, the weight gain goes unnoticed both to the person who is gaining weight and the people who close to that person.

The clothes that we wear do keep getting a little tighter and serve as an intermittent reminder about the creeping weight gain. But we make adjustments to even that reminder When we go out to shop, we buy a size larger than what we had been wearing. Going up a size makes the clothes fit us better. We literally breathe better when we start wearing a larger size of a shirt. This provides a temporary fix to the problem. Once back home, we throw the old, ill-fitting clothes to the back of the closet. The nagging effect that these clothes had on us, also goes away with them, to the back of the closet. The cycle repeats itself every so often and every such time we simply trade in our clothes. In this way, the problem of weight gain is pushed under the carpet.

So what usually triggers self-awareness about weight gain is that one day you meet a friend after many years or try on a pair of jeans from five years back. The friend has a look of surprise on his face when he sees you. The old pair of jeans that fit you beautifully in the past have become so tight you are unable to pull them above your knees.

It is then, that the realization dawns on you, "My God, I am fat!" It might seem at that point that it occurred overnight, but you can see that weight gain of large proportions occurs over many months and even years. The good thing is that the same trigger that makes you take notice of the weight gain can also trigger your quest for weight loss.

Let us look at some statistics from the NWCR. 83% of the participants in the aforementioned study reported that they experienced a trigger that led to their eventual weight loss. Almost 23% had a medical trigger (obesity related medical diagnosis in self or a close someone) that initiated them to lose weight. The other 60% or so had a non-medical trigger that prompted their weight loss. Common amongst these triggers were that they hit a lifetime high of their respective weights, saw an image of themselves (much like I did in the elevator), or wanted to pursue an activity that required them to lose weight. The purpose of mentioning these statistics is to let you know that if you only recently noticed that you are overweight, then you are not alone. It is normal for the weight gain to go unnoticed for a long time. The good thing is, at last now you are ready to do something about it.

CHAPTER TWO

Principles of Weight Loss

Let us get down to brass tacks. There are three interconnected principles that will drive your weight loss.

The overarching of these principles is self-awareness. Self-awareness is what drove you to acquire this book and start reading it. But that is just the beginning. You will need to keep the flame of self-awareness burning to get you through to the other end. I will help you do this by introducing the other two principles of weight loss that you shall be using: daily self-weighing and the use of a pedometer.

Self-awareness about weight loss will drive you to start the self-weighing and pedometer use. Once you start following these two habits, they in turn will keep the self-awareness going. Thus it forms a self-fulfilling cycle.

Self-Awareness

"No one can persuade another to change. Each of us guards a gate of change that can only be opened from the inside. We cannot open the gate of another, either by argument or emotional appeal."
—Marilyn Ferguson, author and proponent of the New Age Movement

External factors and motivators can make a person lose large amounts of weight very fast. However, the effect lasts only as long as the motivator exerts its influence. It is just like a gas pedal in a car. The moment the foot comes off the gas pedal, the car comes to a grinding halt. Similarly, as soon as the external motivator disappears, the weight reappears. Permanent weight loss can only be achieved when the motivation to lose weight comes not from the outside, but from within oneself.

In my own case, the elevator ride that I talked about before was the trigger for self-awareness. It made me look at myself in a new light. I had never considered myself to be fat. I needed a jolt like that to become aware of the reality about my weight. Although that trigger ended once I stepped out of the elevator, it initiated a more permanent realization that I needed to take some action about my weight.

One might think that every person who is overweight would realize their need to reduce their weight. But this isn't so. There are people who are overweight all around who genuinely don't seem to be bothered by it. But are they really happy?

Imagine this scenario. Imagine I had a magic wand and could wave it around and instantly make people lose weight: how many of those people would still choose to remain fat? Not many, I am sure. Given an option, most people would likely cross over to the other side of the weight divide.

People don't need to be overweight. It goes against the very nature of things. When you are fat, your efficiency in every other sphere of life goes down. You can accomplish much less. Imagine a fat deer, if there is any, in a herd. If that herd were to be attacked by a tiger, who do you think would be the most likely prey? The fat one, right? In a primordial sense, a fat human being is as susceptible as a fat deer in a herd.

So, what about those people who appear to be comfortable with their excess weight? Are they really satisfied with the condition of their body? I suspect that they have reached an internal compromise about this. Over time, they have convinced themselves that it is okay to be fat and they start to genuinely believe this. But they need not do that.

Is self-awareness the sole catalyst for weight loss? I am afraid, not, although I do wish that it were that easy. But what it will do is lead you to form habits that in turn will make you lose weight.

Self-awareness acts as a steering wheel that keeps your car on track.

Commitment

Weight loss will only happen when it is your top priority.

Let there be no doubt in your mind about the fact that weight loss requires a deep commitment. This commitment has to be in form of your time, mental space, and even some money. Remember that weigh loss cannot happen externally or passively. You have to take proactive measures to lose weight.

There is no need to be disheartened upon learning that substantial effort is required to shed weight. Yes, initially the amount of time and effort that will be needed shall appear quite daunting. But remember, the human mind and body are very fast learners. They adapt very quickly to the new demands placed upon them. As you start to move along the weight loss journey, the quantum of effort required on a daily basis goes down very fast and weight loss becomes a habit. That is when you reach that state of equilibrium where weight loss is no longer effortful, the point of cruise control, where your foot comes off the pedal but your car continues to cruise ahead. At that point with minimal effort your weight loss is maintained. Your goal is not to go on a special diet and lose ten pounds quickly, only to regain it all back. With these methods, your goal is to develop habits that initially help to lose weight and then maintain the weight loss for a lifetime. You are in it for the long haul.

Let me bring up the car analogy here again. When you're just beginning to learn to drive, every step, like the control of the steering wheel, pressing of the brakes, clutch and the accelerator and their coordination, seems a big effort. Every step requires concentration, effort, and purpose. It seems impossible to do so in the beginning. If you tell a person who is just learning to drive to try and change the radio station while driving, he would think it is impossible. He will tell you, "I can barely keep this thing moving and you want me do something else as well?" Your entire focus is on trying to coordinate the various aspects of driving the car. However, soon enough each movement starts to come more naturally to the novice driver. The coordination needed to manage the clutch, brakes and the accelerator improves steadily. The coordination between the two hands to control the steering wheel and the gearshift becomes better. And then the whole thing starts to come together and it becomes one single, fluid motion. The amount of focus required to drive a car goes down sharply as you become more proficient. And finally the day arrives when you start driving almost at a subconscious level. Of course, you can change the radio stations while driving then without any problem.

This is exactly what is required to maintain weight loss. You will see for yourself that with the techniques described in this book, you will make weight loss into a habit. Once you do that, it will require minimal conscious effort to maintain it.

This is the only scenario that can work on a long-term basis, that of making weight loss into a habit.

I hate to say this, but you have to become little selfish to lose weight. You have to invest time that you might otherwise spend on family, work, or friends. This is because the effort to lose weight comes with strong demands. On a brighter note, much of this extra commitment is required only in the initial period. As it becomes habitual, the amount of effort decreases significantly and you no longer need to be selfish about it.

Benefits of Weight Loss

Losing weight can benefit you on many more levels than just physically.

There is a deeper connection between success in weight loss and that in other spheres of life. Being fat bothers us constantly. It starts bothering us right from the moment when we wake up in the morning. We find it difficult to get up from the bed, literally, because of the excess weight. Every physical movement becomes a strain for a fat person. Getting dressed for the day and looking at ourselves in the mirror reinforces our negative self-image. Our clothes don't fit properly and it's a struggle to even to get into them. By the time we reach our workplace, we are already feeling fatigued. In interpersonal interactions around the office, we are embarrassed to be the largest person in the group. The bothered feeling really never goes away.

And now, reverse this scenario. Look at what happens when we manage to lose weight.

The absence of fat makes us motivated. The paradigm of weight shifts from being a negative force to becoming a positive force in your life.

Let us go through a typical day in the life of someone who was overweight previously and has managed to lose weight. You wake up and literally jump out of bed as you feel more energetic physically. When you look into the mirror you appreciate a much fitter body. The same clothes that you found difficult to get into now fit you very well. You reach your office in a physically fresh state. In your interactions with people around you, not only are you one the fittest people but you are constantly asked how you managed to lose weight. Just as the excess weight was a constant nagging source, weight loss is now a constant positive force in your life.

It is my belief that this is one of the main reasons why successful weight loss can lead to success in other areas of life. It can be attributed to weight loss acting as a constant positive force. I have experienced this myself and seen other people doing the same. Success in weight loss can have an exponential effect in other areas of life.

You don't have to take just my word. Let us look at what the NWCR participants said about the benefits of weight loss. 95% said that their quality of life improved after losing weight. Over 90% participants experienced improvement in their level of mobility, general mood, self-confidence, and level of energy. The benefits extended to their social life as well. A majority noticed improved relations with their friends and coworkers and said that their job performance became better. That's not all. Even their interactions with parents and spouses improved. In short, the benefits of weight loss touched all aspects of their lives.

There is no reason why you can't experience the same thing.

Health Benefits of Weight Loss

I am aware that you have enough motivation to lose weight. Still, I wish to share with you some of the health benefits that would accrue once you lose weight. I also want to mention certain serious health problems that are known to occur as a result of obesity.

Large scale scientific studies provide overwhelming evidence that once you cross a Body Mass Index (BMI) of 20–21, your risk of developing type 2 diabetes, hypertension, cardio vascular disease and gall stones all show a progressive rise. You might have already had some inkling about the association of these conditions with obesity. Now read the really scary part.

Obesity leads to higher chances of you getting cancer. Yes. That is right. Your chances of getting cancer go up as your weight goes up. Every additional 5 kg/m² in BMI in men increases their risk of getting esophageal cancer by 52% and colon cancer by 24%. An equivalent rise of weight in women increases their chances of getting uterine cancer by 59%, gall bladder cancer by 59%, and postmenopausal breast cancer by 12% (the association is strongest in women in the Asia–Pacific region).

Excess bodyweight is linked to people getting enlarged prostate, infertility, asthma and even difficulty breathing during sleep. In fact, you don't even need to be born yet to experience the ill effects of obesity. Maternal obesity has been linked to an increased risk of birth defects in their offspring.

I hope these statistics give you a sense of the serious heath implications of being overweight. The aim is not to scare you but to motivate you.

People are known to get onto the weight loss path after being diagnosed with one of the above conditions. You should not wait for this to happen to you to start losing weight.

Habit Formation

"Most of the time what we do is what we do most of the time. Sometimes we do something new."
—Townsend, D. J., & Bever, T. G. (2001). *Sentence comprehension: The integration of habits and rules.* Cambridge, MA: MIT Press.

I want you to recall a habit of yours. Just one. It should be an action that you do repeatedly, in a similar setting in terms of time and place every time you do it.

Did you come up with one?

How would you categorize this habit? Is it a "good" or a "bad" habit?

Chances are that whatever you came up with, you categorized it as a "bad" habit, rather than a "good" habit.

There is a reason why this happened.

When we think of habits, we usually perceive them with a negative connotation. It could be as innocuous as nail-biting or as harmful as smoking. Whatever the case might be, habits for most of us pertain to whatever we are doing wrong. Most self-help books talk about "breaking this habit" or "getting rid of that habit" (one notable exception is Stephen Covey's *The Seven Habits of Highly Successful People*). The same is true of health information websites. Most talk about strategies to get rid of "bad" habits. Very few talk about acquiring good ones.

It is time to change this thinking.

Habits need not be thought of as bad. There can be good habits as well.

There has been a recent surge in interest about the concept of habit formation and its practical applications in all spheres of life. It is a mammoth concept by itself and I cannot make any claims that I can teach you the entire habit theory in one chapter. It is simply not possible. People have devoted entire books to the subject. If I had to recommend one, it would be Charles Duhigg's *The Power of Habit: Why We Do What We Do, and How to Change*. You will learn almost everything that there is in relation to the practical application of the habit theory.

What I will do, however, is teach you the basics of habit formation in this chapter. And then, throughout the book, I have tried to adhere to these principles in relation to the various habits that can make you lose weight.

What Are Habits?

"First we form habits, then they form us."
—Mark Matteson, author of *Freedom from Fear*

When I set out to find the definition of habits, I found that the medical literature has a multitude of opinions even on this matter. Medical researchers seem to like to individualize almost everything, as per their own understanding of things. This multiplicity of opinions extends to a seemingly precise thing such as a definition!

So, instead of just one, I have chosen a few definitions, in order to cover all aspects of habits in relation to weight loss. You see, I belong to the same fraternity of medical researchers, and would myself like a little variety in opinion, wherever I can find it!

David Neal, a psychologist from the Duke University, defined habits as "learned sequences of acts that have been reinforced in the past by rewarding experiences and that are triggered by the environment to produce behavior, largely outside of people's conscious awareness.

Per Nilsen, a researcher from Sweden, emphasized the "lack of consciousness" part of habits, saying habits are "behavior that has been repeated until it has become more or less automatic, enacted without purposeful thinking, largely without any sense of awareness." If you apply this to eating, you can identify many scenarios, both good and bad, when you eat or drink without any thought. Think of the time you sit with a bag of chips, watching television. It is a classic example of a bad habit in relation to eating. If you recall the last time you did it, you will realize that once you start it, there is no stopping. This is because you get into the "automaticity" mode and are not even thinking or are even possibly aware that you are constantly putting chips in your mouth. Remember the successful commercial for chips, "No one can just eat one"? Well, it appears to me that the makers of this commercial really went deep into the habit psychology and used it to the hilt.

Benjamin Gardner a lecturer of psychology at the University College of London, emphasized "context" in relation to habit. He added the following to the definition of habits: "Behavioral patterns learned through context dependent repetition: repeated performance in unvarying settings reinforces context-behavior associations such that, subsequently, encountering the context is sufficient to automatically cue the habitual response." To simplify things, he said that, for habitual actions to occur, they need a context. And whenever the context is made available to you, you automatically execute the behavior. Let me give an example. Shift workers are used to taking lunch at an appointed hour. Say, a particular worker breaks for lunch everyday at 1P.M. So for him, the clock striking 1PM is the context which triggers his act of taking lunch. Every day at 1 P.M. he will start feeling hungry, wherever or whatever he might be doing. That is the importance of context in relation to habits. These observations have been extrapolated to how we eat. Mark Conner, a psychologist from the Univeristy of Leeds noted that, because eating is something most people do every day and because, in many cases, meals are consumed at the same place and time from day to day, it may be assumed that eating is in a large part habitual.

To summarize, habits have three important ingredients: context, trigger and automatic behavior.

So, something that has been established to be habitual can be effectively changed or made better by changing the habits themselves. There is no other way to do this.

You already have the "bad" habits that made you fat. My aim is to get you to have the "good" ones and lose weight.

How Much of Your Day is Habitual?

"Ninety-nine hundredths or, possibly, nine hundred and ninety nine thousandths of our activity is purely automatic and habitual, from our rising in the morning to our lying down each night."

—William James, American philosopher, psychologist and a trained physician

You might think that habits pertain to some sporadic, specific actions done a few times during the day. We tend to assume that most of our actions are conscious and planned, with an occasional habitual action thrown into the mix. The true picture is quite different.

Let us try a mental exercise.

Visualize your typical day. Start from the time you wake up, and mentally take yourself through the day, step by step. Now try to estimate how many of your actions are governed by habits.

How do we identity an action as being habitual? These are actions that you do almost at a subconscious level or in an automatic manner, without having to think. Let us look at you morning routine in a little more detail. You wake up at a certain time (habit), get up from the bed and reach out for your slippers (habit) and head to the bathroom (habit). There you wash your face (habit) and go into the kitchen (habit). You start a pot of coffee (habit) and go into the porch to get the morning paper (habit). You see how this is going. You can break down any part of the day to identify habitual actions.

So, now tell me what percentage of your actions in a typical day are governed by habits?

What figure did you come up with?

You may not realize it but studies have shown that almost 45% of our actions in a day are committed as a matter of habit. That constitutes an astounding half of our day.

So, when someone tells you "Half the time I wasn't even paying attention," it is probably true in the literal sense, as habitual actions don't require conscious effort on your part. In a way, they occur automatically.

This categorization of half of the day as habitual takes into account all our actions as a whole. If we look deeper into our eating and physical activity, an even higher percentage is governed by habit.

Why Habits Are Important in Weight Loss

"A nail is driven out by another nail; habit is overcome by habit."
—Desiderius Erasmus, Dutch scholar, 1466-1536

If you look at how you gain weight in the first place, you will see that a lot of it is related to habits, "bad" ones if I may add: binge eating, frequent snacking, poor choice of foods. They can also present as a lack of good habits, like not doing enough physical activity. Once these behaviors become habitual, you go on repeating them. And they keep adding weight to your body.

So, how do break out of this vicious cycle? A combination of bad habits and lack of good habits makes you fat. If you can reverse this, you can reverse the weight gain.

Let me bring up the analogy of a diamond here. It is one the hardest materials that is known to man. It is so hard, that you can cut a diamond only with another. A cutting tool made with any other material will fail to cut a diamond. Hence the adage,

"A diamond cuts a diamond."

Similarly, weight gain, which is the result of recalcitrant habits, can only be tackled by cultivating other habits.

Stages of Habit Formation

"Everything you are used to, once done long enough, starts to seem natural, even though it might not be."

Julien Smith, author of *The Flinch*

Habit formation occurs in three stages. First is the initiation phase. In this phase you select the new behavior/habit you wish to adopt, and also decide the context in which it will be done. For example, you decide after reading this book that you want to start weighing yourself daily. So you have "selected" the specific behavior that you want to adopt. The context, has to be defined here. In this case it will be the time between your coming out of the shower and wearing your clothes.

The second phase in this process is the learning phase. In this you start to develop automaticity of the intended habit. Now you start to weigh yourself every day, immediately after bathing and before getting into your clothes. And since you repeat this action in your chosen context (between finishing a bath and dressing), you end up strengthening the context-behavior association in your mind. So, with each repetition daily, you need progressively less effort to remember to weigh yourself. This is the development of automaticity or, using the car analogy, operating on cruise control.

Finally, you enter the stability phase. Congratulations! You have formed the habit!! Its strength has plateaued, and it will stay with you with minimal effort. Now, every day as soon as you finish your bath, you will automatically step onto the scale, almost without even thinking. You will see that it takes very little effort on your side.

A logical question at his point would be, how long does this process take. There is some variability in the time frame required to adopt a new habit. There was a popular idea introduced by the self help literature of the 1980s which states that if you perform an action for 21 days in a row, it gets converted into a habi . I am sorry to burst this bubble. Not only is this an over simplification of the habit-forming process, but it is also incorrect. You cannot establish a habit simply by repeating it; there is more to it. Research in this area has shown that it takes an average of 66 days or about 2 months before a behavior becomes habitual. A good thing is that during this process, the effort required will diminish on a continuing basis. In other words, doing something that is new to you will become progressively easier, until it become a habit, at which point, you will be operating on cruise control.

So, with two months of sustained effort, you will go from "not doing anything" to "doing everything" about your weight.

Keystone Habits

"Remember it is far easier to develop small habits than it is to make major lifestyle changes. You are far more likely to succeed by adding a minute or two of exercise to your routine than you are if you try to commit to an hour of gym a day. Set goals that are so small that it is impossible to fail."

—Akash Karia, author of *Small Habits + Keystone Habits = Big Results! 10 Power Habits That Take 5 Minutes Per Day & Guarantee Rapid Results*

"Once a small win has been accomplished, forces are set in motion that favor another small win. Small wins fuel transformative changes by leveraging tiny advantages into patterns that convince people that bigger achievements are within reach."

—Karl E. Weick, American psychologist and author of *Small Wins: Redefining the Scale Social Problems*

Now that you know how habits work, you should get ready to start adopting new ones and breaking some bad ones in order to lose weight. The smaller the habit, the easier it is to acquire. A small habit that can potentially lead you on to getting bigger habits is the best choice to start with.

The combination of a very small change in your routine and its ability to catalyze other, much larger changes in your life converts a plain habit into a keystone habit.

A keystone habit is a very small habit, that by itself is quite easy to adopt, but it leads you to succeed in acquiring bigger, more complex habits.

There are two keystone habits that I will focus on in this book. The first exerts a big influence on your eating habits, both good and bad. The second will make it possible for you to take up regular physical activity. These two keystone habits will in turn unlock a slew of habits that will make it possible for you to both lose weight and maintain it for a lifetime.

Food/Exercise

There are two variables that determine your weight that are under your direct control.

The first is caloric restriction. You limit your caloric intake by controlling what and how much you eat. The second is increasing caloric expenditure. You do this by increasing physical activity. Both go hand in hand. It may look like straightforward primary school arithmetic at first. Rest assured, if it were that easy, you wouldn't be overweight.

Theoretically speaking, caloric deficit coming from either a reduced intake or an increased expenditure should lead to an equal amount of weight loss. However, long-term studies show that caloric restriction by reducing food intake plays a more prominent role in creating initial weight loss than physical activity. Once the weight loss has occurred, there is a role reversal. Increased physical activity takes the dominant role in maintenance of the weight loss.

There is a mountain of scientific research that says so. The only question left is, how does this happen? Common sense says that it if 3,500 calories equals one pound, howsoever you reach it, it should lead to a weight loss of one pound. It should not matter if you create this deficit by eating less or exercising more. But data shows this isn't so.

Logically speaking, it should not matter where the caloric restriction comes from, whether from dietary restriction or increase in expenditure. Yet it does. Compare these two scenarios. You can reduce 500 calories a day by replacing the 2 cream, sugar filled coffees that you have daily, with plain black ones. To create the same 500 caloric loss by exercise, however, you (let's assume you are a woman, 5"5 tall and weigh 165 pounds would need to run for one hour at six miles per hour. Obviously, the first choice is much more feasible than the second. So, does it mean that if you keep restricting calories, you will keep losing weight at the same rate? The answer is, no.

There are two reasons why the effectiveness of caloric reduction progressively decreases. First, when you reduce your caloric intake, your body is immediately put on guard. As part of evolution, human bodies have developed defense mechanisms to tide over difficult times. So, when you reduce your caloric intake, your body interprets this as a signal of distress. It thinks you are experiencing a famine. So, how does it react? It immediately lowers its resting metabolic rate (RMR) or the calories spent in maintaining itself. And if you remember from the previous chapter, RMR accounts for a massive 70% of your daily caloric expenditure. So, the same body that was spending 1,500 calories a day to keep itself going now goes into economy mode and does the same job with 1,200 calories.

Think of how your laptop computer goes into a power saving mode when the battery level goes down. The same thing happens with your body. By restricting your caloric intake, you are putting your body into a power saving mode. So, now the same caloric reduction of 500 calories a day is effectively is reduced to a reduction of 200 a day, as the body has lowered its expenditure by 300 calories. Hence, the 500 calories you manage to cut out of your diet no longer causes the same amount of weight loss.

Then there is the effect on your body mass. Eating less makes you shed weight. In an ideal world, you would think that all this weight would come from your belly or thighs or whatever part of your body you think could benefit most. What actually happens, though, is very different. Only a part of you weight loss comes from fat. The rest comes from the non-fat part, or mainly the muscle. To make it easier to understand, just remember that fat is lazy.

On the other hand, when you start engaging in physical activity, it not only adds to the caloric expenditure but also does something which is even more important: it brings your body out of its power saving mode. So, now the body starts responding to the caloric restriction again. Thus a healthy combination of the two, caloric restriction and physical activity, keeps your weight in check. There is no doubt, that both are required at all stages of weight loss. It's just that their relative importance changes as you move from weight loss to weight loss maintenance.

We may have learned this after going through tons of research on this subject, but the participants of the NWCR seemed to have already figured this out on their own. It is surely not a coincidence that almost 90% of them modified both their dietary and physical activity habits. The evidence speaks for itself.

Weighing-Food

Weighing yourself daily is the first keystone habit that will help you to adopt eating habits that create/maintain weight loss.

In the NWCR study, 75% of participants reported that weighing themselves at least once a week. Remember, this statistic is from the period when they were in the weight maintenance phase. Presumably, the frequency of self-weighing was even higher when they were actually losing weight.

Why is this so important?

Weight gain happens on a daily, ongoing basis. You don't put on weight by the pound. You put on weight by the ounce. The process occurs in a very gradual manner.

If you weigh yourself daily, you can catch any weight gain that might be occurring in real time. Since the rise in weight depends on your eating habits, more than any other single thing, you get immediate feedback about your eating habits and their effect on your weight.

Once you know how much you weigh, right in the morning, the knowledge stays with you for the entire day. This keeps you aware about your ongoing weight reduction effort. It does not allow you to lose sight of the fact that you need to lose weight. The self-weighing habit has a major effect on your eating habits through the day.

Daily weighing requires a very small action on your part that takes very little of your time. It does not alter your routine in any manner. Also, it does not require any major emotional effort. And yet, it acts a catalyst to much larger habits about eating. Hence, it is a potent keystone habit.

Pedometer- Activity

The second keystone habit that you need to acquire is the use of a pedometer.

A pedometer is a small electronic device, about the size of a thumb-drive, that keeps count of the number of steps that you take. It needs to be worn on one's person in order for it to measure the physical activity that the wearer does in a day.

As with self-weighing, wearing the pedometer itself requires a small, daily physical action on your part. Again, it does not intrude on your routine in any manner. It has all the traits of an ideal keystone habit. It drives you to sustain the requisite amount of physical activity that is required to maintain your weight.

Summary

This is what this book boils down to. I will ask you to make the initial effort to acquire two seemingly small habits, daily self weighing and wearing the pedometer. In the subsequent chapters, I take you step-by-step through the process required to get hold of these two habits. At the same time, you will understand the innate connection of these habits with your eating and physical habits, respectively. As you develop this understanding, you will increase the effectiveness of self-weighing in controlling your eating and that of the pedometer in maintaining your physical activity.

When I was trying to find ways to reduce my weight, I started by using the pedometer as a means to motivate myself to walk more. A little later, I started weighting myself regularly. At that time, I had no inkling about the profound effects of these habits on one's weight. The true ramifications of these habits and their connection with weight loss became clear to me when I stumbled on the NWCR and found that most of the participants were also doing the same. It is then that I realized that what I had been doing, was no fluke. After that I unearthed heaps of medical literature that has shown the benefits of these two habits for someone trying to lose weight. The only piece missing from this puzzle was how these two habits could be used to acquire other weight loss habits. This book is that missing piece

CHAPTER THREE

How to Begin

"The beginning is the most important part of the work." —Plato

How Much Weight You Should Aim To Lose

Do you really need to lose weight?

You need to answer this question scientifically before we proceed any further.

I want to make sure that you are really overweight and are in need of weight reduction. This doubt arises because with the current onslaught of images of underweight models being projected in the media as the "ideal" body types, even people with normal weight might perceive themselves as fat.

I want to ensure that you are not one them.

The simplest way to answer this question is to compute your Body Mass Index (BMI).

You can do it manually on a calculator by carrying out the following steps on a calculator:

1.   Multiply your height in inches times your height in inches.

2.   Divide your weight by that number.

3.   Multiply that result by 705.

Say you weigh 160 pounds and are 65 inches tall. Your calculation will look like this:

4.   Mutliply 65(your height in inches) by 65. You get 4225.

5.   Divide 160 (your weight in pounds) by that number (4225). You get 0.038.

6.   Multiply that result (0.038) by 705. In this case, you get 26.8.

If you don't want to go through this manual method of calculation, you can use one of the online calculators. There are thousands of websites that have tools to determine BMI. I found the one at Centres for Disease Control and Prevention (CDC) the easiest to use (http://www.cdc.gov/healthyweight/assessing/bmi/adult_bmi/english_bmi_calculator/bmi_calculator.html).

Now that you know your BMI, you need to understand the implications. The normal range of BMI is 18.5 to 24.9. So, if you came up with a figure of 25 or above, you need to lose weight.

If your BMI falls in the normal range, you should still read this book as you should be aware of the strategies to maintain your weight and prevent future weight gain.

Anything less than 18.5, makes you seriously underweight and you actually need to put on weight. In this case, please gift this book to someone whom you think is really fat!

How Much Weight To Lose

Your first target should be to "normalize" your BMI.

If you used the CDC website for BMI calculation, you may have noticed that it gives you the range that your weight should fall into. So, for the previous example, it gives the normal weight range as 111 to 150 pounds (for a person weighing 160 pounds and with a height of 65 inches). This person needs to lose just over 10 pounds, to enter the "normal" weight category. He or she could, however, choose to lose up to almost 50 pounds and still be in the normal weight range. However, 10 pounds is the minimum amount of weight to be reduced for such a person.

You can set any target weight that you like yourself to weigh in the end, the only condition being the target weight should place your BMI in the healthy range, i.e. 18.5-24.9. As long as your target weight is in this range, you are good to go.

Now You Have A Target

Once you have calculated the minimum amount of weight that you should aim to lose, you have achieved a transformative thing. You have converted an abstract desire, of wanting to lose weight, into a well-defined goal. No one has said it better in the context of importance of setting goals than Tony Robbins, the famous life success coach and author of *Awaken the Giant Within*. He says, "Setting goals is the first step in turning the invisible into the visible."

By putting a concrete number on the amount of weight that you need to lose, you have turned an abstract dream of losing weight into a concrete target.

Put The Weight Loss Equation To Work

I know you want to lose "a lot of weight, very fast." I wanted the same for myself when I made up my mind to lose weight. Everywhere you look there are books and websites that are selling dreams along the lines of, "lose 10 pounds in 2 weeks" or "shed 30 pounds in a month". As a result, when we do resolve to lose weight, we start thinking in terms of a couple of weeks or a couple of months simply because we have been conditioned to do so.

But as I found out and you will too, significant and long-lasting weight loss does not happen in few weeks or even a couple of months. One thing is certain: you cannot achieve weight loss that is safe or permanent over the course of a couple of weeks. To experience weight loss that is safe and lasting, especially when you are talking about tens of pounds of weight loss, that requires many months, or even more.

Let us look at some facts before we decide how "fast" you can lose weight safely and reliably.

For every pound of weight you want to shed, you need to create a negative caloric balance of 3,500 calories. This is an irrefutable fact and any weight loss (loss of body mass and not just loss of water) has to adhere to this law. There is no going around this fact, so wrap your mind around it. The sooner you do it, the better off you'll be.

Say you want to lose ten pounds. To do so, you will need to lose a cumulative of 35,000 calories (10 X 35,00 = 35,000). It is an established fact that people can create a negative caloric balance of 250-500 calories per day without needing special diets or medical supervision. A daily deficit of more than 500 calories per day needs to be supervised by a physician, to be safe.

So, with a caloric deficit of 250-500 per day, you will need 70-140 days to accumulate a loss of 35,000 calories (70 days if you are creating a negative balance of 500 calories per day and double of that or 140 days if you are reducing daily caloric balance by 250).

This translates to a weight loss of one pound a week (at 500 calories/day) or one pound over two weeks (at 250 calories/day).

This is a universally applicable calculation and you can apply it in any setting where you need to check the safe rate of weight loss. You can see quite clearly that the fastest you can go is one pound of weight loss every two weeks. So there is no question of losing "10 pounds in 2 weeks" or other promises of this scale.

Simply put, those claims are hocus pocus and nothing else. So do not waste your time dreaming about losing many pounds of weight in a couple of weeks.

CHAPTER FOUR

Self Weighing:
The First Keystone Habit

"I have been struck again and again by how important measurement is to improving the human condition."

—Bill Gates, Founder of Microsoft

In my early days of weight loss, I started to weigh myself regularly. At that time, I did it only out of curiosity. I wanted to see for myself the outcome of my efforts. I had no inkling at the time that this habit itself drives the weight loss process. I started doing it to check how much weight I was losing. The fact was that regular self-weighing itself fries the weight loss process. Slowly, as I began to notice that my weight was going down, I also got into the habit of noting my daily weight in a notebook. This was the start of the formal daily weighing process that I refined later on.

At that point, I had not grasped the significance of this seemingly small habit. I knew it was pertinent to my weight loss efforts and kept on doing it, but I had not understood that in fact, it was the regular self-weighing that was helping me to lose weight. It was later, when I learned about the NWCR and came to know that most of the participants in that were also weighing themselves very regularly, that a light bulb wen off. I became conscious of the fact that there was more to it than was initially apparent. Subsequently, when I came upon medical literature on this subject and analyzed studies on the role of daily self-weighing, I put two and two together and figured out the connection between daily self weighing and weight loss success.

Daily weighing keeps you in a constant feedback loop. On days that you stray and end up eating a lot, the consequence shows up immediately the next day. You will compensate for your indulgence once you see its result. And over a period of time, the repeated effect on your weigh-ins as the result of binge eating may help to keep you away from such extravagances.

You should make this into a daily habit and try and not miss any days of measurement, especially after the days when you slip up, where the urge to skip a weigh-in is greatest.

Daily self-weighing will take only two minutes of time every day. However this will be the linchpin that holds the entire bridge together. It's the most leveraged single action that you can undertake in your effort to lose weight because it will have a cascading effect on your day.

Self-monitoring has been studied extensively by researchers, who have found conclusively that weighing yourself daily is most likely to lead to weight loss as compared to less frequent weighing, including weekly and monthly intervals. Further, if you weigh yourself daily, you are more likely to retain the weight loss over long-term periods. Some people imagine that daily weighing may somehow cause psychological problems. Relax. Scientists have studied this aspect of daily weighing and they have found that daily self-weighing is not associated with any adverse psychological symptoms at all. So lay your doubts to rest about it.

Go ahead and start weighing yourself daily and maintaining a record. It will help you to lose weight, maintain the weight loss and make you exercise even more! A win-win situation!

Buying Your Scale

You should invest in a reliable and robust weighing scale. It will be your partner in the weight loss journey.

There are some important aspects you should keep in mind when you are buying a weighing scale.

It has to be a digital weighing scale. If you are still stuck with a traditional version with the analogue scale, it is time for you to discard it. It just won't fit the bill. With the precision required for regular self-weighing, you definitely will need to buy a digital machine. Further, the new machine should give the readout of the weight in one-tenth of a pound.

The machine needs to be accurate and consistent. If you are buying it in a physical store, it is easy to check for accuracy. Place the machine on a hard surface (avoid putting it on a carpet). Step on it, and note the reading. Come off the machine and weigh yourself again. The second reading should match the first reading exactly, down to the tenth of a pound. If it does not do so, don't buy it. Period.

Another feature that you should consider is the body fat percentage measurement. However, things are not as simple as measuring the body weight. The currently available weighing machines meant for regular consumers are almost as accurate and consistent as the ones used in scientific studies. As far as body fat measurement goes, these machines have a long way to go before they match up with the machines and techniques used by scientists. To be fair, I must mention here that the gold standard for such measurements that can pass the scientific muster require that you be immersed in water, fully, in order for the measurement to be accurate. There is no way that a normal person can be asked to that! So we take the next best thing, which are the consumer-grade weighing machines with the body-fat measurement feature.

The test that you did to check the weighing accuracy won't work with the body fat measurement. You will have to be a little lenient here. In any case, if you will be measuring body fat percentage regularly, I will ask you to rely on weekly averages of such readings and not just the daily measurement. This will minimize the day-to-day variations. We will be relying upon the absolute percentage value of the body fat measurement. Rather, we will be observing the trend in measurement. And, if you measure yourself in a consistent manner, almost any machine will be able to give you a trend of the body fat percentage accurately.

Recently, scales have started coming with a nifty little add-on feature. They can be connected through your home wifi to dedicated apps for phones. This is a useful addition that can help you to keep track of your weight. It takes away the task of manual recording your weight and there is no limit to what an app can do with the data.

It does take a little effort to get the machine to "talk" to your phone, but once configured, it generally works quite well. The manufacturer Withings was a pioneer in these type of machine.

And now, Fitbit also has it's own version of a wifi-enabled weighing machine called Fitbit Aria. I am a little biased towards the Fitbit version as it integrates well with its phone app.

There are lots of fancy looking machines which are made to look very sleek. Don't make that a factor when buying a weighing machine. Sleekness should not be a consideration when buying a weighing machine. You should look for something that is actually heavy. It will be more stable when weigh yourself, and hence will probably be more consistent. When it comes to sale, size does matter and the bigger, heftier machines are preferable over the sleek, slimmed down versions.

Establishing Baseline

The first step in the self weighing process is to determine your true baseline body weight and body fat percentage.

Let me explain why I use the term "true" here.

A single weight reading is not an accurate refection of your current weight. This is because every instance of weight measurement is influenced by factors like the time of the day, food/drinks intake on that day, your clothes. Even the alcohol that you might have taken the previous day can affect your weight the next day. Since the baseline weight is going to be an important anchor in your weight loss journey, you need to be accurate. Only then, will your subsequent efforts would truly be comparable.

Since we will rely on the weekly average of your weight readings (average of your last seven weight readings), you will need to spend the first week creating the baseline. So, in the first week, go about your activities as you would normally do. Try not to alter your eating or activity patterns. Also make sure that you are not travelling out of town that week.

A good time to start weighing yourself is on a Sunday. This way you can get a true snapshot of your body weight through the entire week.

Now you need to fix the time of the day when you will be weighing yourself everyday. Since you eat differently through the day and will have varying hydration as the day progresses, the best time to weigh yourself is the morning. I prefer to way myself right after my bath and before I get into my clothes. In this way, I manage to standardize a lot of conditions for the daily weigh-in, including clothes (as I am wearing none!), food intake (I am usually empty stomach as I eat my breakfast after taking my morning shower) and the hydration status is pretty constant as I usually have had a cup of coffee before the bath. Another benefit of following this routine is that I have slotted the time at which I weigh myself between coming out of the bathroom and dressing. This is a crucial step, as the finishing of the bath is the "cue" that leads me to weigh myself. This way, I never forget to weigh myself daily.

"Your first ritual that you do during the day is the highest leveraged ritual, by far, because it has the effect of setting your mind, and setting the context, for the rest of your day."
—Eben Pagan, American business entrepreneur, author and speaker

The early morning weigh-in acts as the first domino in your daily routine, setting in motion the rest of your actions in relation to food and physical activity. Once you have your daily weight reading, it sets the tone for the day.

Since this program requires that you weigh yourself daily, I want to use the preparatory week in establishing your weighing routine. See what works best for you. Try to get into the groove of measuring your body weight in a standardized manner and truthfully every day. Also you will see that when you actually record figures daily in a tabular form and can easily comapre the readings of the preceding days, it serves as a powerful reminder of the current status of your weight. And as you become used to weighing yourself every day and, more importantly, recording it, you'll see that this simple action serves as a very effective self-check mechanism.

Weighing Process

Once you have your baseline weight established, you can continue to weigh yourself daily.

Every day, get on the machine once and weigh yourself.

To get into the habit, it is important to fix when you do this. The "when" is the context that is the part any habit. In this case, I recommend that the context is the period between your coming out of the shower and before dressing. Once you start doing it, you will see that it starts to become an automatic process.

Weight Log

Keep a small diary and pen next to the scale. Record your weight and body fat percentage in the diary every day.

Use the following steps for creating your weight log. Make a table and have three columns it. The left column is for the date. Write the dates of the entire month in that column. The middle column is for your weight. The right column is for your body fat percentage.

There are several advantages of recording your weight in this manner. When you write your weight in a table that has space for the entire month's record, any day you miss doing it will show up as a blank space. This blank space serves as a reminder for you to be more consistent in weighing yourself daily.

When you log the day's weight, you will tend to look at your measurements over the previous days. At this point, two things happen simultaneously. First you'll compare your weight that day with that of the previous day. If you have been good with your regimin, it usually shows up as a loss of weight in a day. But if you have been undisciplined and have binge eaten, it will definitely show up as a significant weight gain. Although a part of this gain is temporary in nature because of water retention, seeing the number will make you more likely to make amends the next day. The memory of this will also help you to control your urge to eat the next time you are in a situation where you otherwise might end up binge eating.

The second effect is that you also get a sense of the general direction in which your weight is headed. For example, if your weight has been hovering around 160 pounds throughout the month, it means it has been steady. However, if you notice that at the start of the month your weight was lingering around the 160s and but now the readings are 161 pounds over many days, you can be sure that your weight has increased.

Thus logging your weight gives you both a daily and a monthly overview of your progress. This dual mode of feedback is very effective in keeping you on course.

Concerns About Weighing Daily

There is a concern amongst some people over the concept of daily self-weighing. One of the most vocal arguments was raised by Michelle Dionne and Fiona Yeudell in their article "Monitoring of weight in weight loss programs: a double-edged sword?" They wrote "daily self weighing may generate negative states and increased body dissatisfaction, which can ultimately undermine weight loss efforts."

These are potentially serious repercussions and need to be addressed adequately so that there is no room for any doubt

When you look at the fine print of these studies that raise concerns about the potential ill-effects of regular self-weighing, a different picture emerges than what come up on cursory reading of these studies.

All these studies were conducted amongst normal weight, non-treatment seeking individuals. This greatly limits the implications of these studies. Moreover, in two of these studies participants were purposely given inaccurate feedback regarding their weight. They were either told they were 5 pounds heavier or lighter than they actually were. This greatly complicates the issue and fails to bolster the argument against self-weighing. Further, none of these studies produced any evidence that self-monitoring one's weight causes body dissatisfaction.

Paradoxically, regular weighing has been valued by many of the participants of these studies. Many said that they liked the accountability that comes from regular weighing because it helps them maintain focus on their dietary and exercise efforts in the face of adversity. Scientific literature is consistent in its conclusion that regular monitoring of body weight is associated better weight control in the short and long term.

Weight monitoring allows you to notice how specific situations or patterns effect changes in body weight. Because you are recording yourself daily, it is easy for you to remember what you ate or did the day before. If you went out for a party and gorged on a buffet meal and the next day you find that your weight has jumped up by a pound, you will automatically realize the deleterious effect of binge eating. This way you can learn to identify specific actions that affect your weight, both in a negative or a positive manner. There is no need to think that it is only intended for negative feedback. It also provides an opportunity for positive reinforcement when certain behaviors produce a desired result.

Frequent self-weighing can increase dietary vigilance and thereby help to maintain successful weight loss. Consistent and more intensive self-weighing can allow you to catch weight gain before it escalates. It facilitates weight control by enabling you to catch and divert small weight gain there and then.

In studies on self-weighing and weight loss, it was found that participants who decrease their self-weighing frequency end up increasing the percentage of caloric intake from fat and decrease in their ability to control their eating habits. Conversely people who increased the frequency of their self-weighing experienced less weight gain. So any way you look at it, daily self-weighing can help you at many levels in both losing weight and maintaining weight loss.

One has to guard against laxity in the daily self-weighing routine. Research has shown that the initial high level of adherence to self-weighing is followed by a gradual decrease. And if you drop your guard in the frequency of self-weighing , your weight will start to creep up again. The only way to counter this is to make it into a habit. You will be encouraged to know that these same studies showed that self-weighing was perceived positively, and as easy to remember.

Benefits of Daily Self-Weighing

Researchers from Duke University conducted a study called Weighing Everyday to Improve and Gain Health (WEIGH). (Health researchers seem to have a fetish for jazzy acronyms, and this is as good as it gets, for a weight related study!) The main purpose of the study was to investigate the relationship between daily weighing and other weight control behaviors. At the beginning of the study, the researchers hypothesized, "based on self regulation theory, daily weighing would lead to greater adoption of weight control behaviors." Simply put, they wanted to know whether daily self-weighing would lead to adoption of other weight loss habits. Participants in the study were instructed to weigh themselves daily using a special electronic scale that was provided to them by the researchers. The scale was modified so that it automatically transmitted its readings to the investigators in real time. The participants were provided with tailored feedback and skills training via weekly e-mail messages about habits that would lead to weight loss. By using these special scales, the investigators were able to objectively measure the frequency of self-weighing. They also measured various diet, exercise, and behavior-related outcomes associated with weight loss success.

Although all the people in the study were given the same instructions, only some of them succeeded in weighing themselves on a daily basis. Others did so less frequently. So, in order to determine why this happened, the two groups groups were compared.

The results of the study were striking. After six months, the daily self-weighers managed to lose an average of 20 pounds while the non-regular weighers lost a little less than seven pounds. Even though the second group weighed themselves almost five times in a week, they fell short of the daily self-weighing requirement.

The difference between weighing themselves five times a week versus seven times a week, though not seemingly significant, was enough to cause a 13-pound weight gap between the two groups. This finding was no fluke. Daily self-weighing was found to have influenced many weight-related habits, which in turn led to much greater weight loss. Both eating and physical activity were seen to be affected. Those who weighed themselves daily reduced their snacking between meals, reduced the frequency at which they ate out at restaurants, reduced the frequency or portion sizes of their desserts, and eliminated high-calorie foods from their home or office. By adopting these habits, the daily self-weighers reduced their daily caloric intake by 600 calories, compared to a reduction of 353 calories for the less frequent self-weighers.

Their physical activity habits improved too. The daily self-weighers reduced the amount of television they watched, exercised daily for a period of 30 minutes of more, and increased the number of steps they walked.

Who could imagine that a seemingly small habit like stepping on a scale could lead to such drastic changes in behavior? And yet it did. It appears from these studies that self-weighing acts like a yoke, keeping our weight under tight control.

A word of caution: Don't be tempted to think that simply by weighing yourself daily, you will lose 20 pounds in six months. Weighing by itself doesn't do anything to the weight. It is a keystone habit that will lead you to adopt other habits in relation to eating and activity that, in turn, will make you lose weight.

To summarize, daily self weighing leads to progressive weight loss. However, what happens once you do reach your target weight? Do you need to continue weighing yourself daily?

This question has been answered nicely by a group of researchers from Tampere University of Technology, Finland and the Cornell University, working together.

They studied the relationship between the frequency of self-weighing and the weight changes in a group of people who needed to lose weight. Specifically, the researchers wanted to examine the effect that breaks in self-weighing had on the peoples' weight. The participants in the study were asked to weigh themselves daily and were given advice about weight reduction for eight weeks. They were then left on their own but were asked to keep weighing themselves. The investigators wanted to see how meticulously the participants kept up the routine and what effect the regularity of their weighing had on the weight.

A strong relationship was found between self-weighing frequency and weight change. During the period in which the participants were weighing themselves regularly, their weight decreased consistently. When, they became inconsistent in weighing themselves, though, the weight slope reversed and they started to gain weight.

Interestingly, the researchers found a sweet spot at which the participants' weight became constant. This occurred when they weighed themselves every 5.8 days or approximately one week. So, when they weighed themselves once a week, they neither lost nor gained any weight. Just what you want when you are in the weight maintenance phase.

Those whose weighing frequency fell to once a month or even less ended up gaining weight.

Does this finding sound familiar? What the researchers found in 2014 was already known to people in the NWCR for many years. This group already weighed themselves once a week during their weight maintenance phase.

What does this mean for you?

During the initial phase, when you are trying to lose weight, you should aim to weigh yourself daily. Once you reach your goal weight, you can drop the weighing frequency to once in a week. However, be vigilant. Anytime you notice your weight creeping back up, go back to daily weighing. A practical tip for knowing when to go back to daily weighing is when you notice that your weight has crept up two pounds. That is the time to switch gears and ramp up the weighing frequency from weekly to daily weighing. Any complacency in this will take you further away from your ideal weight. And the farther off you veer, the harder it becomes to return.

So, daily weighing for weight loss, and weekly weighing for weight maintenance, is the mantra.

Possible Pitfalls and How To Avoid Them

One scenario when you might miss weight measurements are the days when you're traveling. I don't recommend using weighing machines in hotels to do this job. It is the consistent weighing that is important. So even one pound difference between the machine at your home and the one at the hotel will unnecessarily spoil your weight chart. One pound lower measurement on the hotel machine will push you to eat more during your trip and a pound more on the hotel machine will unnecessarily demotivate you. So just make sure that you weigh yourself immediately before leaving home for the trip on your own machine and also the day you return. Any laxity in terms of sticking to your weight equation during the trip will immediately show up on the machine and you can get back on track of weight loss.

Another problem to watch out for is the fact that scales that measure body fat run out of batteries sooner than regular scales. Keep a set of extra batteries handy for the machine. You don't want to miss a couple of days of measurement just for the want of batteries.

Also be aware that the body fat measurement may be influenced by the moisture on your feet. Ensure that you dry your feet before getting on the scale.

In terms of frequency, weighing yourself once a day is enough and in fact preferable to weighing yourself every time you pass by the scale. Intraday fluctuations may unnecessarily disturb you. Also, weighing yourself once a day creates a sense of anticipation and uplift. You can lose this energy if you keeping yourself multiple times during the day. It is like knowing the result of a game before it even starts. It ruins the pleasure of watching the game.

Finally, for the scale to give accurate results, always keep the machine on a hard, stable surface. Never keep it on carpet. This is especially true of a machine measuring body fat, which must be kept very stable.

Self-Weighing and Caloric Intake

Every instance of self-weighing affects your dietary and physical activity habits in more ways than you can imagine, but the effect is more pronounced on your dietary habits.

The first thing that weighing yourself does is make you aware that you are engaged in a weigh loss process. Much like when we are driving long distances, we can fall asleep, we can lose sight of the fact that we are trying to lose weight. In fact, there are devices available on some cars that monitor your wakefulness, and can jolt the seat with vibration or even emit a mild electrical current in the steering wheel if it detects that you are falling asleep. Weighing yourself does exactly the same thing. The most direct effect of weighing yourself is that it keeps you "awake" in your weight loss journey.

The next thing that happens is that it motivates you. Comparing the day's weight to the previous day's leads to one of the two following outcomes. The day's reading is lesser than the previous day's weight. It instantly gives you positive feedback. It tells you that whatever you did the previous day was effective in keeping your weight in check. Or, the day's reading is higher than the previous day's weight. Again, you get instant feedback, but this time it is cautionary. So, gradually, it will also start curbing your overeating instincts.

Food

In the 1980s, Robert Crandall, former chairman and CEO of American Airlines, was trying to look for ways to cut running costs in his company. Amongst other things, he noticed that a green olive was being served as a garnish on the salads served to the passengers. After making a few back of the hand calculations, he calculated the total number of meals being served to passengers on the American Airlines flights every year. He estimated, that by eliminating one olive from the meals served to the passengers, the airline could save $40,000 per year. He also guesstimated that eliminating a single olive would go unnoticed by the passengers, and therefore would not cause any collateral damage in the form of customer dissatisfaction.

The airline implemented the idea and managed to save over $40,000 the next year, just as Crandall had predicted. The story has since become business folklore, cited by management gurus.

There are two important lessons to learn from this story.

First is that to be viable, any change in your eating habits has to be very small and subtle. It should be so small that it almost goes unnoticed by you. Crandall chose to eliminate only an olive from the salads as it was unlikely that flyers would notice its disappearance. Imagine if he had tried to substitute something like a steak with some thing cheaper or even removed it from the menu altogether. Sure, it would have had a much larger impact on the bottom-line than the elimination of a single olive, but would it have gone unnoticed by the paying passengers? Most certainly not. The reason that the missing olive went unnoticed was that it was a very small change. The meal experience would have remained almost the same with or without the olive. You will be playing the same trick with your diet, that of trying to make changes that are so small they go unnoticed by you, and yet which are significant enough to reap rewards.

The second lesson from this artfulness was that, even a small change, if carried out over a long period of time, can lead to big benefits in the end. If someone were to say that a single olive can cost $40,000, it would sound implausible. Yet, this story shows how it can be done. Similarly, every calorie that you eliminate from your dietary intake will add up and lead to substantial weight loss.

Both these lessons will form the crux of your endeavor to adopt better dietary habits.

Now let's find your $40,000 olive.

Believe me, there are more than one hiding on your plate.

Getting an Estimate of your Current Caloric Intake

I've heard a lot of people say, "I don't eat that much, and yet I keep on gaining weight." Are you one of them?

In most cases, this perception arises from your inability to accurately take into account all the food that you eat through the day. If you are going to try and reduce the number of calories that you consume, it is vital that you first have an accurate picture of how much you are eating.

When you are asked about your daily food intake, the natural response is to take into account the major meals of the day and probably some snacks that you might remember eating. The problem is that even if you are accurate in accounting for these major meals, you still may not be getting a true picture of your actual food intake because we tend to discount certain foods we eat. Not only do these "hidden" foods increase your daily caloric intake, but they are also more difficult to control because they are not even on your radar.

Examples of such hidden foods are: the many bites you take to test the food while cooking it, the packet of lozenges or gum that you consume, that "one" cookie that you eat with your sugarless coffee, and many such things. I bet if I ask, "How much food did you eat yesterday? you will not account for every item. This is the prime reason that most of us have an inaccurate estimate of our actual caloric intake.

The only way to detect these hidden sources of extra calories is to create a food log. You can do this by hand or with one of the many smartphone apps. The idea is to capture everything that you eat or drink throughout the day, howsoever small or inconsequential it may appear... even the fish oil supplement that you might be taking everyday. (By the way, each capsule of fish oil supplement has about ten calories!) Yes, it is a cumbersome thing to do. But is quite feasible if I ask you to do it only for a couple of weeks, maximum. The idea is to get a fairly accurate, baseline picture of your caloric intake. And since you will be only making small changes to your dietary habits, you will not need to create food logs later on.

To accomplish this, keep a small notepad with you throughout the day. Whenever you eat or drink anything, write it down in the notepad. In order not to miss anything, make sure that you have noted the previous food eaten before you eat anything else. In this manner, you will not miss anything. Only plain water is exempt from this. Everything else that you eat or drink, without exception, goes in the notepad. Also note the quantity ingested. This can be in the form of an exact measurement in weight or volume if you are eating from a packaged product that has a food label. If, however what you are eating does not have a nutrition label, like a self prepared item, remember to note the quantity either in unit form, e.g. " 2 slices of bread," or an approximate measure, e.g., "a cup of milk."

At the end of the day you should have a log of you entire caloric intake. Now, what remains is to calculate it. For this, many websites are available to do the job. My own favorite is calorieking.com. It is a very comprehensive site and lists almost all possible food items, including branded foods.

Once you calculate your total daily caloric intake, the figure you come up with might be a real shocker. There is a common refrain that I have heard a lot from people who are trying but failing to lose weight. They think that they are eating much less and exercising much more than they actually are. Most of them blame their "genes" or "slow metabolism" for their inability to lose weight. In their minds they are doing all the right things and yet are not managing to lose weight. Most have already either thrown in the towel or are ready to do so. I would probably do the same if I were in their position. But there is a catch.

Are they really doing what they say they are doing or is their perception off? Do you also belong to this group?

A National Institutes of Health funded study published in the New England Journal of Medicine (NEJM) in 1992 debunked this perception.

They recruited a group of overweight people for the study,

separating out a group of eleven people who were suffering from "diet resistance," that is, claiming that they were eating less than 1,200 calories every day and yet were unable to shed any weight. The other group consisted of 80 people who also had failed to lose weight but who knew they were eating too much.

Both groups were studied very closely over the next 14 days. The scientists carefully measured actual caloric intake and expenditure of these people, during this period.

If the claims of the "diet resistant" group were anywhere close to truth, their measured caloric intake should have been found close to 1200 calories a day.

The results of the study were surprising. Not for the scientists, but the people in the "diet resistant group."

During the 14 days, when every calorie that they ate was measured diligently, it was found that they were taking in about 2,100 calories a day. This observation made it clear that they were underestimating their caloric intake by almost 50%. They were not victims of "diet resistance." They were simply not expending as many calories as they were consuming, just as is the case with every person who becomes fat.

The second group of people consumed about 2,400 calories a day, but thought that they were taking in about 1,700 calories. So, they were also under-reporting their caloric intake, although only by around 20%. Fair enough. There will always be some discrepancy between how much food we perceive we are eating and how much we actually are. In fact, every overweight person tends to underestimate their caloric intake.

This study punctured the myth that many people have about

the apparent discrepancy between their eating habits and weight loss efforts.

If you also think that you are consuming less calories than your weight has to show for it, it may just be a case of underestimating your caloric intake.

Keeping an honest food log, just as the people in the NEJM study did, can help clear any doubt you might be harboring about your food intake.

Although I have outlined how to get a fairly accurate estimate of your caloric intake by keeping a food log, that is not its only purpose. The other is to make you aware of your eating habits. When we are asked to estimate how much we eat daily, we tend to remember only the major meals. In my own experience, what we eat in our major meals – breakfast, lunch and dinner – usually does not play a major role in making us fat. These meals are usually regimented in terms of what and how much we eat. Of course, if you eating lunch in a restaurant, this is a different matter.

It is what we eat in between these meals when we snack that really impacts our caloric balance. The unpredictability of snacks goes a long was in contributing to caloric imbalance: the fact that the food itself can vary, and that the timing and frequency of the snack can vary. The food log helps us to identify these apparent blind spots in our thinking about what we really eat through the day. A carefully kept food log can uncover many such eating habits that we might not even realize in a normal course. This to me is the biggest benefit of keeping a food log. Once you identify the small things that you eat in between major meals, you can quite easily work on eliminating them.

Setting a Caloric Reduction Target

Once you have an estimate of your daily caloric intake, the next step is to determine the deficit that you need to create in order to lose weight.

The US National Institutes of Health's clinical guidelines on obesity recommends that a caloric deficit of 500 to 1,000 kcal/day be prescribed as an integral part of a weight-loss program. 500 calories a day adds up to about 3,500 calories a week or one pound of weight. The maximum caloric deficit that you can safely sustain is 1,000 calories a day, amounting to 7,000 calories a week, which would result in a weight loss of two pounds in a week. This calculation shows that with dietary control, you can safely achieve a weight loss of one to two pounds a week.

It should be amply clear to you by now that whatever you may do, the maximum rate of weight loss that you can hope to achieve is two pounds in a week. Advertisements that claim that you can lose up to ten pounds in two weeks are unrealistic. As you can see from the simple calculations above, losing anything more than two pounds a week is not feasible, especially on your own.

The next logical question is, if you create a caloric deficit of 3,500 calories per week, will you keep on losing a pound a week in perpetuity? No, it does not work like that. This is actually fortunate, otherwise a 150-pound, calorie-restricting woman would disappear completely in 75 weeks.

To understand why the weight reduction effect of caloric deficit drops over time, imagine you start at a weight of 150 pounds. At this level, let us say that your daily caloric requirement is 2,000 calories. If you consume 2,000 calories a day and maintain your usual level of physical activity, your weight will remain stable. Now, you wish to lose weight and go on a diet that that provides you 1,500 calories a day, 500 calories short of your daily requirement. Initially, you will manage to lose about one pound a week. Now, assume that you lose 15 pounds in 15 weeks and now weight 140 pounds. Will a 1,500 calorie diet produce a weight loss of one pound a week? No, it won't. This is because when you weighed 150 pounds, your body required 2,000 calories a day to sustain itself. At that weight, a 1,500 calorie diet produced a caloric deficit of 500 calories. Now, when you weight 135 pounds, your caloric requirement has also dropped by 10% (you have also lost 15 pounds or 10% of your body weight). So, now your daily caloric requirement is less by 10% or 1,800 calories. Hence, if you continue to consume 1,500 calories a day, you are now creating a deficit of 300 calories a day. So, now with the same diet it will tale almost 12 days instead of seven to accumulate a caloric deficit of 3,500 calories. Hence, now you need almost two weeks instead of one to lose one pound of weight.

As you can see, when your weight drops, so does the rate of your weight loss, owing to metabolic adaptations in your body. One such adaptation is a reduced metabolic rate. This occurs as a result of decreases in metabolically active tissue or in hormone concentrations. Second, the energy costs of daily activities are lower at reduced body weight. Say you weigh 150 pounds at the start of your weight loss journey. At this point, your BMR would be approximately, 2,000 calories per day. If, however, you reduce your weight to 135 pounds or by 10%, everything else remaining same, your BMR will also drop by 10% to 1,800 kcal per day. Therefore, in order to continue losing weight at the same rate, you must also gradually reduce energy intake to maintain a constant negative energy balance. To do this, the caloric deficit should follow the reduction in caloric requirements at lower body weight.

Even if you are not sure about your total daily caloric intake, you can still set a caloric deficit goal. You can do this by simply deciding your desired rate of weight loss and then reducing your calorie consumption at the rate of 3,500 calories per week to target losing one kilo every two weeks without even calculating the baseline.

How does Food Make you Fat

Your perception about food and its role in making you fat has to be centred on the fact that you need to consume 3,500 extra calories to put on 1 pound of weight. If you look at it carefully, you'll find that 3,500 calories is actually a lot. Even the largest meal you might have eaten till today may not reach the level of 3,500 calories.

Let me give you a few examples.

Imagine the most fattening foods you can think of. Take a one-liter tub of ice cream. Even if you were to eat the entire tub, you would be surprised to know that you would be adding 2,000 calories to your diet. You actually need to eat almost two full tubs to put on one pound of weight. Surprised? Now consider pizza. Sometimes after a particularly large pizza binge, you are almost sure that you have put on at least a couple of pounds of body weight. Now consider this. A large pepperoni pizza packs 3,000 calories. Even if you were to eat the whole pizza, you would still fall short of gaining even a single pound.

My purpose is not to condone binge-eating. Rather, I want to demonstrate that an occasional excess in eating does not contribute much to weight gain. It is the regular intake of extra calories that is the real culprit. Let us look at another example. Assume that you have a habit of eating a cookie with your morning coffee. The label on the packet says,claims it has very low fat and high fiber. You look at the nutritional information and notice that a single cookie has 70 calories. This doesn't sound like much, especially in comparison to things like ice-cream and pizza. But consider the long-term implication of eating this cookie on a daily basis: over a period of a year it would add up to 25,550 calories. This equates to a potential gain of over seven pound of weight. If you compared the weight-gaining properties of pizza and cookies in isolation, you would pick pizza every time as the food more likely to cause weight gain. But as this example shows you very clearly, it is the habit of eating certain things that make weight gain more likely.

If you look back carefully at your eating habits you will be able to identify not one but many such habits. All of these are potential targets for you to hit. If you can find them, you are in luck.

Eliminating such seemingly small habits is actually quite simple. The difficult part is locating them. You tend to notice the big ticket items, the cakes, the pizzas, the steaks and in the process the small, but equally important food habits slip under your radar. You can identify such habits by simply keeping a food diary, albeit only for a couple of weeks,. I know it is very tedious and impractical to keep a food diary on a very long-term basis. It simply cannot work. But if you know that you have to keep a food diary for only a couple of weeks, I think you may find it feasible. A food diary will help you identify things like a cookie eaten with your morning coffee or that piece of chocolate or cheese that you eat after dinner every night. It is these seemingly small things — the ones that slip past your radar – that add up to very large sums of calories over long-term.

What You Eat

Mathematically speaking, if you eliminate 100 calories from your daily diet, either by choosing not to eat a cookie that has 100 calories in it or by walking 45 minutes and burning 100 calories, both should have equal impact on your weight.

But that is speaking in the mathematical sense.

In the real world, things work a little differently.

A huge mass of clinical studies has proven beyond doubt that for weight loss to occur, caloric reduction by way of dietary restriction is more effective than reducing calories through physical activity. However, once you have lost weight and are trying to maintain it, the role of physical activity usurps the role of diet.

A word of caution here. Don't think that physical exercise plays no role in weight loss or that you don't need the support of good dietary habits in the weight maintenance phase. It is not a black and white system. No, certainly not. Both are required, only their relative importance reverses in the two phases, dietary restriction in the initial reduction phase and physical activity in the maintenance phase.

Named Diets

Diet literally means "the kind of food that a person habitually eats." Yet today, if you were to hear the word diet, chances are you would construe it as a reference to caloric restriction.

It is usually never, simply diet. When we think of the word "diet" we usually add an adjective to it, "vegan diet", "gluten free diet" "low-carb diet".

Diet has mistakenly come to be associated with something that is out of the normal.

One possible reason for this spurious mental association, especially by someone who is trying to lose weight, is the explosion of "diets" for weight loss over last few decades.

Almost everyone has heard of these diets and they all seem to carry some sort of magical aura about them. So why not start with something that is "magical"?

I thought that it would be best for you if you learn the principles behind these diets, their relative efficiency in making you lose weight and why they are apparently successful in doing so.

The most important reason however, is that I want you to understand why they often fail at some point.

We have something to learn from both their successes and failures in weight loss.

Any special diet that is designed to make someone lose weight has a dietary principle at its core. This principle is usually one of the following two: either being a low-carbohydrate diet or a low-fat diet. Regardless of the fancy names that some commercial diets carry, the truth behind them boils down to one of these two principles.

Has some of the sheen already started to come off? And I am just getting started.

Any food that you eat is a combination of carbohydrates, proteins and fats (and water, which plays a negligible role here).

From a nutritional standpoint, foods differ only because of the difference in the relative proportions of the three main constituents.

The named diets, all of them, recommend juggling these proportions.

Examples of low-carbohydrate diets include Atkins, South-Beach and Zone diet. They caution that no more than 40% of your caloric intake should come from carbohydrates. The rest of the caloric intake can come from a combination of proteins and fats.

Ornish and the lesser known Rosemary Conley diets fall into the category of low-fat diets. These focus on restricting your fat intake. If you follow one of these diets, fats should account for less than 20% of your daily caloric intake. As with the low-carb diets, the rest of your calories are split between the two remaining constituents. In this case, fats and carbohydrates.

Commercial weight loss programs like the Jenny Craig, Nutrisystem,Volumetrics and Weight Watchers lie somewhere in the middle. They want you to restrict both carbohydrates and fats in moderation.

If you noticed, all the diets focus on restricting either the fat or the carbohydrate intake. No one seems to mind the proteins.

There is one big takeaway that I want you get from this. As far as weight loss goes, fats and carbohydrates are the components to restrict in your diet. Proteins are your friend.

Edward J. Mills and his colleagues from the Stanford University, compared the relative efficiency of famous diets in producing weight loss. They included results from all the diets that I have mentioned above.

They found that six months after being on such diets, participants on low-carbohydrate diets lost an average of 19 pounds and those on low-fat diets lost about 18 pounds. A difference of about a pound. When these people were tracked for a further six or twelve months, the good effects of their dieting started to wane. The low-carb group had regained about three pounds and the low-fat group managed to put on about one and a half pounds. The good effect of these diets peaked at six months from the time people started following them. From there, things went downhill.

There are two lessons to be learned from this study.

First, any special diet intended to cause weight loss will make you lose weight, provided you follow it. The quantum of weight loss is also almost similar across various diets. You can expect to lose about 18 pounds in 6 months, provided you follow the prescribed diet meticulously.

At the end of the day, the caloric balance is making you shed weight and not some magic. In one way, this finding establishes the fact that the weight loss equation is all pervasive.

The other message from this study is that diets only work as long as you follow them. In the Mills Study, after one year, the effect of eating special diets on weight loss had gone down by 10-17%. And this downturn happened when the participants were still supposedly following their respective diet plans. It is not difficult to guess what would happen once they went off these diet plans. Almost all the weight that had been lost would likely be regained over a period of time, and maybe even some more.

So, any diet can help you lose weight, but only as long as you are willing to follow it. You stay with a diet plan, you keep losing weight. You go off it, and the weight returns. That is the story of special diets.

The question I ask you here is, how long do you think it would be possible for you to follow an artificially proportioned, low-carb or low-fat diet?

Can you follow any of them for life?

CE Finley from the Cooper Institute in Dallas tried to answer this question when he studied the Jenny Craig Platinum Program and assessed how long participants stuck with the plan.

Over a one year period in 2001-2002, he evaluated more than 60,000 people who joined the program and found that more than half of the new customers dropped out within three months of joining. And by the end of the first year, almost 94% had left the program. Only 6% remained in the after one year.

A 6% retention rate after one year. Digest this fact.

I expected the retention rate to be low, but certainly not this low.

To give the Jenny Craig people their due, some of the participants might have left because of having achieved their weight goals. But it would only account for some of the dropouts, certainly not all of them. Even people from Jenny Craig would have to agree on this.

The exact reasons for people leaving the program were not available to the researchers. They did, however, propose some potential reasons, including cost, scheduling conflicts/travel, and tiring of the food.

Data from other commercial weight loss programs also shows high attrition rates, albeit of varying degrees.

One thing is certain though, all the major commercial weight loss programs based on diet modification suffer from high attrition rates.

What should you make of these facts? Instead of following any one of these diets, you can pick up key principles of eating from each program so that, although you may not eat solely according to one of these plans, you can incorporate certain specific, beneficial eating habits inspired by them.

Energy Density

It is very easy to tell someone to eat less in order to shed weight. No one knows about the futility of this advice more than you. Your inability to adhere to this advice probably got you here in the first place.

There exists a dietary principle that can bring you out of this rut. This principle is known as the energy density of food. It is a powerful concept that can help you control your caloric intake, without having to resort to starving yourself. It is one of the major tenets of eating that helped me to lose weight.

It's utility lies in the fact that it can help you control your caloric intake, and yet has very little overt effect on the volume of food that you eat. It is one the highly leveraged activities in the weight loss arsenal, and can provide results that are disproportionately high in comparison to the effort that is required.

Energy density is the amount of energy in a given amount of food, expressed in calories/grams.

To make it easier to understand, recall the school science question, "What weighs more, a pound of cotton or a pound of iron?" As you may recall, both weigh the same. The volume of the two, however, is very different. While you would be able to hold one pound of iron in your hand hand, a ball of cotton weighing the same would probably take up half a room. This is the essence of the concept of density.

Let us look at a real world example in relation to food to better grasp both the concept and the utility of energy density in relation to weight loss. Consider the example of popcorn and potato chips. One cup of potato chips weighs about 28 grams and contains 150 calories. On the other hand, one cup of popcorn weighs only four grams and has just 15 calories. Six cups of popcorn are required to match the weight of one cup of potato chips. And even when you compare these quantities, popcorn still has only 100 calories, compared to the 150 calories contained in one cup of potato chips. To match them calorie for calorie, you would need ten cups of popcorn to reach the figure of 150 calories contained in a single cup of potato chips. In terms of calories, one cup of potato chips has the same number of calories as in ten cups of popcorn. It is quite easy to see where this is going. Eating ten cups of popcorn will definitely make you feel much more fuller than eating one cup of chips, although you will end up consuming an equal number of calories.

That is the power of energy density of food.

Let's delve into this a little deeper.

Calorie content is just one aspect of food. How full you feel after eating any food determines how much of it you will end up consuming.

To test this, researchers from ConAgra, owner of the popular brand of ACT Popcorn, conducted an experiment. They recruited 35 healthy people as test subjects. The volunteers were given one of three different snacks on three consecutive days: either one cup of popcorn, six cups of popcorn, or one cup of potato chips. Half an hour after eating the test snack, the participants were offered a meal consisting of mac and cheese. They were asked to eat as much mac and cheese as they wanted. After three days, the exercise was repeated with a different snack followed by the same mac and cheese meal. On another day, they ate the mac and cheese meal without any preceding snack, to serve as a control group.

By knowing the amount of mac and cheese the participants eventually ate after each type of snack, the researchers could estimate the satiety each of the test snacks had caused. The fuller a test snack made a participant, the less mac and cheese they would eat.

The researchers found that participants experienced less hunger and more satisfaction with a snack of six cups of popcorn compared to when they ate one of the other test snacks or even when they had no snack. Further, the total caloric intake including the calories in the snacks and the mac and cheese was significantly higher when they ate potato chips than when they ate popcorn.

As you can see, the energy dense snacks like chips do very little to make you feel full, but they do end up increasing your total caloric intake. In comparison, snacks with less energy density satisfy your hunger more effectively and end up making you eat less. This is the leveraged action capability I was talking about, of achieving satiety while consuming less calories.

How do you identify foods with less energy density?

Two components of food have the maximum energy lowering effect: water and fiber. The more water and fiber in your meal, the less energy density it will have.

On the other end of the spectrum are fats. They have the highest propensity to increase the energy density of a meal. Fats by themselves have the highest energy density amongst all food classes at nine calories per gram. So, fats like butter or oil in a dish greatly increase its energy density.

The question is, how can you use these principles to lower your caloric intake?

Water has zero calories and hence is the best option to reduce calorie density of any dish. The formula to reduce energy density of what you eat is simple, increase the water content and reduce the fat content. Since a major part of satiety comes from the spices and condiments in the dish, watering it down and increasing the spices will maintain the taste while bringing down it's energy density. Vegetables and fruits are a great surrogate for water. Most vegetables have 80-90% water content. Hence by adding them to any dish, they can increase its water content without the need to thin it further with water. You can even use this strategy while selecting food in a buffet. For example, if you are eating pasta, instead of just putting pasta on the plate, choose half pasta (high energy density) and half vegetables (low energy density). You will still enjoy the pasta and will have reduced the energy density on your plate by almost half, as vegetables like tomatoes and celery have almost zero calories. I have given a list of some of these vegetables at the end of this book, that add almost next to nothing in terms of calories to your meals. I call them "free foods" as they have practically no calories.

The other strategy of decreasing energy density is fat reduction. This is little trickier than the previous trick.

If you are cooking food yourself, this is a little easier to do as you have control over what goes in a dish. In this case you just have to reduce the oil or butter in the dish by a quarter or a third to bring down its energy density. You will hardly notice any change in the taste or the flavor of the dish if you do this.

However, if you are eating out, controlling energy density becomes more challenging and it may not be feasible to alter the fat content of a dish. What you can do is remember the fact that oily or buttery dishes will have a higher energy density than others. Look for descriptions like baked or steamed on the menu. Selecting those dishes will reduce the energy density of your food intake. Restaurants do tend to serve dishes that are very high on the energy density score. A typical meal out in America has almost double the number of calories compared to a meal at home. Specific strategies to prevent excesses while eating out are covered in greater detail in a later section.

Another approach that can help you lower the energy density of your overall meal is to eat a portion of low density food like salad or a thin soup before eating your main course. This can help you to lower the final energy density of your meal, thus reducing the total caloric intake.

Barbara J. Rolls from Pennsylvania State University has done major work in the area of food density and weight loss.

She headed a study that measured the effect of eating salad as a first course before a high energy density meal of pasta.

Forty-two women participated in the study. They were asked to eat varying amount of salads before eating as much pasta as they liked. The study found that when the volunteers ate a large portion of a low density salad as the first course, they ended up consuming almost 100 calories less in total after having eaten the full meal. Importantly, when they were asked to rate their liking of both the salad and pasta, they gave equal marks to both the dishes. This strategy is very easy to implement and can yield significant benefits in terms of caloric reduction.

I used this technique extensively when I was trying to lose weight. At that time, I didn't know that there was scientific research behind it. I just applied logic. You, however, are now aware that this is based on solid science and should have more motivation to follow it.

One reason that the concept of reduction in energy density can be adopted as a habit is that it does not require you to change the ingredients of what you eat by much. The application of this strategy requires you to slightly alter the consistency of the dish while maintaining the basic taste. This can easily become habitual, as it does not disturb your long settled dietary preferences.

Compare this with the changes that you need to make while following diets such as Atkins, which asks you to eat only certain types of foods and completely avoid others. Now that is difficult to follow for a lifetime. Adding extra veggies or some water to your next dish is a much easier habit to adopt, even for a lifetime.

Awareness About What you Eat

You have to develop an awareness of the nutritional composition of whatever you eat. You don't need to be precise down to the last calorie or accurately measure each gram of fat or protein in a burger, but you do need to have a fairly decent idea about the caloric content and relative nutrient composition of whatever you eat. It sounds a difficult thing to do, but believe me once you start practicing it, you will learn it very fast. And soon it becomes a cinch.

The first step is to start reading food labels wherever possible.

There are a few things that you should look for on a nutrition label. The first is the number of calories. Typically, the label on a packaged food/drink mentions the calories per serving. Note that in most cases that particular food or drink will have more than one serving. Hence, number of calories per serving can be misleading. Take a two-liter bottle of Coke for example. The label says 140 calories per serving. The critical part is that the bottle has six servings. So, everything that you see on the label, has to be multiple by six in order to know the nutritional value of the contents of the whole bottle. So, the bottle as a whole has 840 calories. This is what you should know because on most occasions you will estimate how much you end up consuming from container as a proportion of the bottle and not by the serving sizes mentioned on the container. So, if you end up drinking about half a bottle, you would have consumed around 420 calories. This is the awareness that you need to develop. You should become aware of the amount of calories in the entire package and not just per serving.

The other thing to note is the amount of protein and fat mentioned on the label. Again, you should be computing the amount of protein and fat in the entire package and not just per serving.

Carbs/Fats/Proteins

Energy from food comes from three major individual food classes: carbohydrates, fats and proteins. Each component has an important role to play in how our body functions. However, our weight, or more specifically, our weight loss and maintenance, depends on the respective proportions of each of these three food classes in our meals. All the special diets that are out there, the low-carb, low-fat, high-protein and others, juggle around these proportions. The goal of each diet is nevertheless the same, to help you lose weight.

As a student of the Weight Loss Habit, there is no escape from grasping the importance of this proportion-juggling act. Once you understand this, you will be able to apply vital nuances from many of these diets to your dietary habits. Since I will ask you to adopt only the core principles from these diets and not follow any diet in particular they are more likely to stick with you for a lifetime, as habits.

The relative importance of carbohydrates, fats and proteins in the diet, with respect to weight loss, was identified in a very cleverly designed experiment by a group of Danish researchers in 1999.

They recruited a group of 65 overweight men for the six-month long study. These men were divided into three groups.

The men in the first group ate a high protein diet so that 25% of their daily caloric intake came from proteins.

The participants in the other test group ate a high carbohydrate diet and only 12% of their daily caloric requirement was met by proteins. Both test groups were, however, asked to restrict the fat content in their diets to a level where no more than 30%. Participants could eat as much as they wanted, there being no restriction on the caloric intake, as long as they adhered to the relative proportion of carbs and proteins in their meals. The third group carried on with their normal diets and served as a control group, a group whose diet mirrored that of a normal population.

After six months, the three groups were compared.The group that ate a high protein diet lost an average of 20 pounds in just six months. Almost 17 of these came from their body fat. The group that was given high carbohydrate meals also lost weight, although a much lower amount of 11 pounds.

Remember, both groups had restricted their fat intake to a similar low level and the "juggling" was done with the proteins and carbohydrates and there was no restriction on the total amount of food that they could eat. They ate as much as they wanted, provided that they maintained the relative proportions of the three food classes in their meals, as per their group classification. Also, they followed their old routines in all other aspects.

The third group, who were not asked to make any changes, showed no change in their weight.

A couple of things become clear from this experiment.

If you restrict fats in your diet, you will lose a certain amount of weight, irrespective of whatever and how much you eat otherwise.

Second, if you increase the proteins in your diet while keeping the low-fat part intact , you will experience an even higher level of weight loss.

This is the crux of the food habits that you need to adopt: reduce the amount of fat that you eat and increase the amount of protein. Manage to do this and you will lose weight, no matter what.

Proteins

The Atkins diet is not a fluke. Its basic requirement is that you reduce your carbohydrate calories to 5-10% of your total caloric intake while at the same time increasing calories from protein to 40-50%. Contrast this with the caloric intake of an average American, only 12-15% of which comes from proteins.

By itself, the Atkins diet can be quite effective in helping you lose weight. Sure, if you follow it, you are almost guaranteed to lose weight. The problem is that it stops working the moment you stop following it. And truth be told, you will stop following it at some point because it asks you to make drastic, almost unnatural changes to your diet.

There are, however, lessons to be learned from this diet, as it is based upon certain valid scientific principles. We may not follow the Atkins diet to the last letter, but we can surely use some of its tricks, and those we can hope to keep for a lifetime.

The main pillar on which the Atkins diet rests is the high protein intake. As you read this section, you can discover for yourself why a high amount of proteins in your diet can make you lose weight.

Increased Thermogenic Energy

The food that we eat needs to be processed by the body to yield energy. The processing part itself uses up a percentage of the calories contained in that particular food item.

Consider a power plant that uses coal to produce electricity. However, as you would imagine, the power plant itself uses up certain amount of electricity in order to function. In the same manner, our body expends some amount of energy goes to process the food we eat.

Proteins are the least energy efficient in that sense. 20-30 % of the energy contained in proteins is used up by our own metabolism. Carbohydrates require 5-10% and fats 0-3% of the energy contained in them for their own processing by the body. This means that eating proteins gives you a discount of 20-30% on the amount of calories, right off the bat.

If I were to use the car corollary here, fats are the most efficient fuel of the three food classes, with only 0-3% of the energy contained in them being spent on their metabolism. Proteins on the other hand, are the "least" efficient fuel because 20-30% of their energy gets spent producing energy.

For someone who is trying to lose weight, the more wasteful the fuel, the better it will be as it will lead to the lowest caloric intake. Hence, proteins are the best choice for weight loss as 20-30% of the calories contained in them don't "stick"' to your body.

Effect on Appetite

The other major mechanism by which proteins help you is by having a higher effect of satiety. In other words, calorie for calorie, compared to carbs and fats, proteins will satisfy your hunger more effectively. So, if you eat a dish with a higher proportion of proteins, it will make you feel fuller earlier, and for a longer period of time. This is the second "secret" behind the success of high protein diets in managing to reduce weight.

Preservation of Resting Energy Expenditure

Even when you are completely stationary, your body is still burning calories just to maintain itself. This is known as the Resting Energy Expenditure (REE).

This is actually a very cool thing, almost utopian, for a person trying to lose weight. Imagine: your body is burning calories while you are slumped on your couch watching TV, or even while you are sleeping.

However, this expenditure can vary a lot.

So what determines your resting energy expenditure?

A major determinant of your REE is your body composition. The muscles and fat that make up the body burn up varying amounts of energy at rest. Fat is the culprit here, again.

Fat is lazy in a sense. A kilo of muscle burns about ten extra calories per day as REE compared to one kilo of fat in the body. The difference may not appear very significant at first. However, it can have big benefits.

Let me explain.

The resting energy expenditure is a "free" pass to burning calories. It operates in the background. You might compare it to the concept of passive income. You build an asset like a second home, lease it to tenants, and the income keeps on accruing. The same is true of REE. For every kilo of fat that you replace with muscle, your body burns an extra 10 calories per day. You literally don't have to move an inch to get that extra burn.

Now let's expand the example. Say you gain about ten kilos of muscle. That translates to 100 calories of "free" burn everyday, calculated at ten calories for every kilo of muscle. This will amount to 3,000 calories per month and 36,500 calories a year. And remember, these extra calories are coming from burning fat. So, at the end of the year, the extra 10 kilos of muscle will burn 5 kilos of fat on their own. Now, do you see the significance?

How does protein fit into this?

Well, increased protein independently increases the muscle mass in the body.

How much Protein to Consume

If you consult research studies on the relationship between protein quantity and weight loss, the consensus is that you have to incorporate 1.2-1.6 grams proteins per kg body weight in order to see its effects. So if you weigh 70 kgs, you would need to consume about 84-122 grams of protein daily. These figures are indicative only and just intended to convey the concept. I don't want you to sit with a kitchen scale at your next meal trying to measure the amount of protein. The bottom line is that you really need to work in raising the protein content of your meals in order to reach the necessary levels.

I myself did this by choosing protein-based dishes or by preferentially picking up protein rich constituents from dishes. A good practical example is when you are eating chicken pasta. It has three major components, chicken, vegetables and pasta itself. Instead of blindly serving yourself, practice a little bit of mindfulness here. Serve yourself the maximum amount of chicken and vegetables thereby increasing the proportion of protein in your serving. The higher their proportion, the better it will be from weight control point of view. The idea is that you should look to increase the protein component of your meals whenever possible.

Increasing the Protein Intake

If you are a meat eater then increasing protein in your diet won't be difficult. Most meat has a very high proportion of protein. Depending on the type of meat, it may contain almost 20-40% protein by weight. You should choose lean cuts whenever possible as this will cut down on the fats that come as a part of any meat product. Looking at the preparation aspect, the best options to cook the meat are broiling, roasting, or grilling. Again, these types of preparations will limit the fats in the dishes. Meat eaters are at an advantage here as they can easily hit their daily protein requirement in only one or two meals by eating meat.

If you eat eggs, then again you will find it quite easy to fulfill your daily protein requirement. Each egg white contains 4 grams of the highest quality, pure protein. In fact, quality wise, the protein in an egg white is so good that it is considered the reference protein by biochemists and is given a score of 100. You may consider egg whites to be almost a "free food" in the sense that you can almost eat them as much as possible with little downside to both your health and weight. Just be careful of one thing. Don't end up adding oil or butter. When I say "free food," I mean egg whites in boiled or poached form.

For vegetarians, things are a little trickier. Most vegetarian sources of protein have a lower concentration of proteins than meat. In order to compensate for this, you need to increase both the volume and frequency of your protein intake.

The top vegetarian sources of proteins include: Beans/Lentils (20%), Whole grains (7-10%), Nuts (20%) and dairy products (5%). Soy products are one of the few vegetarian products that can rival meat in terms of their protein content. Almost 40% of soy beans are protein. So, if you like soy bean products, try and incorporate them into your diet.

Unlike a non-vegetarian diet, where one or two meals can provide enough protein for the day, vegetarians have to incorporate protein in all their meals. But you will soon find that once you start actively looking for protein sources, you will find them almost anywhere.

Fats

There are really only two things that you should be looking to cut down in your diet. One of them is fat and the other is added sugar. I will be discussing fats in this section.

Understand one thing, fats can actually make you fat. The mechanism by which they do it is exactly opposite to how proteins help you lose weight. Fats increase the energy density of foods as they have the highest number of calories per gram of any food constituent. Second, by virtue of being a very efficient food in terms of metabolism, with only 3% of the calories in them going towards their metabolism, 97% of calories from fat go into your body's account. If this were not enough, they also have the lowest potential for providing satiety or fulfilling your hunger. So, if you are eating something rich in fat, like fried snacks, you will almost definitely overeat as your body won't realize the amount of calories it's consuming.

All this makes one thing clear: you will have to reduce your fat intake in order to lose weight. To do this, first identify your sources of high fatty foods and then go after cutting them down. The top sources of fat are oils, butters, cream and animal fat. The way they get into your diet is mostly through cooking. So the best way to cut down fats is to avoid adding them to your meals. Also, try and stay away from things that are fried. Another significant source of fat is packaged foods. Identifying and hence tackling them is a bit easier. Read the label! Always check for the amount of fat in a given package of food and remember to calculate the fat in the whole packet and not just the fat in one serving.

This is one habit that you will have to work on. But remember that participants of the NWCR all adapted themselves to consuming low fat diets. So this is something that can be turned into a habit for a lifetime.

Sugars

If you want to lose weight but still consume added sugar in you food and beverages, well, you just won the weight loss lottery. Added sugar is one of the easiest foods to target for weight loss.

Sugar makes you fat by two primary mechanisms. Sugar-sweetened beverages, like colas, although carrying a significant amount of calories, provide very little satiety or any type of feeling of fullness. Drinking a cola might take care of your thirst, but it will not do anything for your hunger. If you drink a cola with your meal, the calories from the cola will just add on to the calories in the food, because by themselves the sugars in the cola won't do anything to satiate your hunger. In other words, they are "empty" calories.

Sugars are also quite fattening because they have high energy density. Think of cakes, cookies, and ice cream. Most sugar rich food packs in a very high amount of calories per gram.

Combine the high energy density with low satiety index, and you get a potent mixture of fattening foods.

As per the National Health and Nutrition Examination Survey (2005–2008), an average American consumes approximately 21 teaspoons of added sugars daily. At 16 calories per teaspoon, that equates to a caloric load of 336 calories every day, just from added sugar. That is why I consider this a low hanging sweet fruit (pun intended) in matters of weight loss. It is a huge problem and hence presents an equally big opportunity.

The easiest sugars to target are those added to beverages like tea and coffee. Since you add them on your own, it is in your control. In my own experience, I found that if you are used to adding sugar to your beverage of choice, then you will find it difficult to adjust to the taste if you go cold turkey and stop using sugar all together at once. This goes against our basic principles of habit creation. A better way to do this is to reduce the sugar gradually. To do this, start by halving the amount of sugar per serving. If you find that the taste gets altered too much for your liking, then reduce it only by a third initially. You will see that a part in reduction in sugar quantity does not alter the taste of the drink too much and makes it easier for you to adjust to the lowered sugar. And soon the lowered sugar level becomes your new normal. Once it reaches this point, reduce it further, and eventually you will reach a point where you are putting either very minimal sugar in your beverages or even none at all. This is a really easy way to cut down on your caloric intake.

The next source of added sugar to target is the stuff that's hidden in beverages like cola. Most people do not realize the amount of added sugar in sodas. A 16-ounce bottle of Coke has 11 teaspoons of sugar in it. Here we are, trying to reduce sugar by half a spoon at a time and here comes a single bottle of Coke, with 11 teaspoons of sugar. Do you see the absurdity of the situation? There is no way that you can justify to continue drinking sugared sodas. On one hand, they are loaded with sugar calories and on the other, they are without nutritional benefit. If you're used to having them regularly, you need to either stop abruptly or start looking for alternatives, but there is no way that you can continue drinking those drinks and still be in the weight loss game. The best alternative is plain water. It is the perfect zero-calorie drink. If you prefer, you can add some variety by trying sparkling water or even fruit flavored water. Other options are things like 100% fruit juice. They do have calories in them but they are much less than in the sodas and at least do have some nutritive value. Then there is the option of "diet sodas." It is a controversial topic by itself. Like many other issues relating to diet and weight loss, researchers have not been able to decide whether to explicitly recommend them or caution against their use. The best-case scenario would be to restrict or even not drink the diet sodas, but if you do have to have them, then they are a better option than sugared soda.

One thing I would like to caution you about is the "healthy fruit juices." A lot of them come with either added sugars or have a huge quantity of innate sugar. Fortunately, all of them come with nutrition labels. Always check the label for the sugar and calorie content. You may be surprised by what you see. Look around and go for the option with the least number of calories.

Alcohol

The world consists of two kinds of people: those who drink alcohol and those who don't. If you belong to the non-drinking group, you may safely skip this section. However, if you fall into the other group, please continue reading.

Alcohol drinking is an extremely divisive issue. Even while I was looking at medical literature during the research for my book, this divisiveness stood out prominently. In most areas relating to obesity, researchers seemed to take one side or the other, but things were different when it came to the relationship between alcohol and obesity. For reasons beyond my understanding, most researchers seemed to tiptoe around this topic, without formulating a clear message.

I will also not take a side on the issue, since it is an emotive topic and I don't want to be judgmental. Instead, I will lay out some of the major issues in relation to alcohol and obesity. Then, you can make up your mind about what will work best for you.

Are you still reading? O.K., then I can safely assume that you drink alcohol and are trying to lose weight at the same time. I have both good and bad news for you.

Let me break the bad news first. Alcohol impedes your weight loss efforts in more ways than you can imagine.

There are three ways in which alcohol affects your caloric intake.

First is the caloric load of alcohol itself. Each gram of alcohol contains 7.1 calories. In real world measures, every pint of beer has about 180 calories and a double measure of spirits like vodka, whiskey, gin, each have 110 calories. These are all considered to be "empty" calories, nutritionally speaking.

Second are the mixers with which spirits are typically mixed, like cola and juice. In addition, most cocktails include some amount of sugar syrup. Depending on the type and volume of the mixer used, an equivalent amount of calories are added to the existing caloric load of the spirit itself.

The third way in which alcohol affects caloric intake is less obvious, as it is indirect. It has a significant impact on your food intake, both during and after drinking alcohol. This concept will require a little more explaining.

Light to moderate drinking (less than 30 grams of alcohol, or about two small measures of spirits or one pint of beer) does not seem to be associated with obesity in most studies. However, drinking more than this or binge drinking is most certainly associated with obesity.

And this is if you are drinking straight up, without any mixers. The problem with alcohol is that usually, you will not have just one drink. You will have a number of them, so multiply the number of calories in each glass by the number of drinks you usually have. And this is just the start. Alcohol drinking is usually accompanied by some forms of snacking. To compound the problem, in most cases these are the extremely energy dense snacks like peanuts, chicken wings, potato chips, and similar things. And as you become intoxicated, you lose self-control over your eating and drinking and keep consuming more and more. We are still not finished yet with the impact of drinking on the calories that you ingest.

Have you noticed how hungry you feel after drinking alcohol? Not only does it stimulate your appetite but it also makes you lose control over your eating. So you end up stuffing yourself with food after you have had alcohol. And that is not the end of story. After a night out, where you have had a lot of alcohol, the next morning you might wake up with a bad hangover. A casualty of the hangover is that you end up missing your exercise routine for the day.

There is one piece of good news. If you do drink alcohol, consider that you have hit the mother lode of weight loss. It is one of the lowest hanging fruits that you can find. If you do become motivated to cut down on alcohol or even eliminate it totally from your life, you will have discovered a very easy method to cut out a lot of calories from your diet. If you drink once a week, four times a month and cut this by half you are getting a benefit of a calorie cut of around 3,000 calories per month. That is hundreds of calories per day just by making an adjustment on two days. Now that is one of the most leveraged acts that you can undertake to limit your caloric intake. Think about it.

Vegetarianism

Like alcohol, vegetarianism is an emotive and potentially divisive topic. People tend to feel strongly either for or against it. As I did with alcohol, I will play the Swiss Neutrality Card again here and won't take any sides. I will lay out the facts, though, and leave it to you to decide.

The Academy of Nutrition and Dietetics is the world's largest organization of food and nutrition professionals. Founded in Cleveland, Ohio in 1917, it was dedicated to helping the government conserve food and improve the public's health and nutrition during World War I. At the time of writing this book, the Academy has over 75,000 members drawn from a wide pool of registered dietitian nutritionists, dietetic technicians, registered, and other dietetics professionals holding undergraduate and advanced degrees in nutrition and dietetics, and students, in effect, everyone who is qualified to speak on what we should or should not eat.

Fortunately for me, they published a position paper on vegetarian diets in 2015 and hence made my job much easier.

I will share with you some key points from this paper.

The first thing they do in this paper is clarify what a vegetarian diet, because there seems to be some sort of a confusion about this. A vegetarian diet is a plant-based diet that is devoid of all flesh-based products. Note that this definition does not exclude dairy products or even eggs. Other diets like vegan, macrobiotic, ovo-vegetarian and some others, are sub-types of vegetarian diets. All of them are plant based diets, with some individual variations amongst them.

Now coming to the operative part of their judgment.

They take the following stand: "It is the position of the Academy of Nutrition and Dietetics that vegetarian diets may provide health benefits in the prevention and treatment of certain health conditions, including atherosclerosis, type 2 diabetes, hypertension, and obesity. Well-designed vegetarian diets that may include fortified foods or supplements meet current nutrient recommendations and are appropriate for all stages of the life cycle, including pregnancy, lactation, infancy, childhood, and adolescence. Vegetarians must use special care to ensure an adequate intake of vitamin B-12."

What does this mean to someone like you who is trying to lose weight? There are two points to consider here. The first is that vegetarians weigh less than those who are omnivorous. That is true at the baseline level. What if you are omnivorous at present and were to turn vegetarian? How would that affect your weight? Well, that question was answered by a study from George Washington University School of Medicine. They compiled results of other major research studies that had evaluated the effect of becoming vegetarian on body weight. They found that on average people lost 410 pounds each just by becoming vegetarian. Remember that there was no caloric restriction by these people, the only thing that they did was turn vegetarian and they ended up losing significant amounts of weight. There were two distinct mechanisms described in this study that can explain why this happened. The first is that vegetarian diets in general are high in fiber and are low in fat. This in turn lowers the energy density of food consumed by vegetarians compared to that eaten by omnivorous people. You already know that reducing energy density lowers you caloric intake which in turn reduces tour weight. The second mechanism is a little more convoluted. It is thought that vegetarian food has a higher thermic effect on caloric burn as compared to meat-based foods. Simply put, your body puts in more effort to digest vegetarian foods than it does for meat, and thus fewer calories end up in your system. The only caveat that everyone seems to agreeon is that if you turn vegetarian, you must take some form of Vitamin B12 supplementation. All other nutrients, including proteins, are well taken care of by a vegetarian diet.

I rest my case here.

Becoming vegetarians is not simply a matter of adopting new dietary habits. It is a profound socio-cultural change for someone who has been a meat-eater. I have stated the facts about a vegetarian diet and its effect on weight. It is up to you to decide what you would like to do in this regard.

Final Lesson on What To Eat

In real life, you can't be expected to weigh every meal or analyze every dish for its contents. This is not possible nor do I want you to attempt it. Constant, overly critical analysis of what you eat can rob you of the simple pleasures of life that come from eating.

So, how do you enjoy food and still manage to lose weight at the same time?

After having understood how various elements in food make you gain or lose weight, you start to identify foods accordingly. Simply put, there are things that can positively affect your weight loss and things that can negatively affect it. As you learn to identify them, you will slowly start to increase the good foods and decrease the bad foods. As you will understand with time, you can apply multiple principles of intelligent eating to every meal.

To summarize, remember that proteins should be consumed and fats should be avoided. Carbohydrate-rich foods should lie in the middle of your priority list. You should try to drastically reduce or even eliminate all forms of added sugars in your meals and drinks.

Try and apply the concepts of low energy density wherever possible. This is easily done by adding extra water to dishes when feasible and increasing the proportion of water-rich vegetables in dishes.

You should consider the issues of alcohol consumption and vegetarianism.

How You Eat

We now move on to the second aspect of eating: the "hows" of eating, as it pertains to the various situations and times when you eat food and how you can learn to adopt better habits of doing so.

If you think about it, it is much easier to modify the "hows" of eating than the "whats" on a long-term basis.

Breakfast

"Eat breakfast like a king, lunch like a prince, and dinner like a pauper"
—Adelle Davis, nutritionist and advocate of unprocessed food and vitamin supplementation

One of the crucial findings of the National Weight Control Registry (NWCR) was that 78% of the participants ate breakfast every day. This finding has profound implications.

In addition to weight loss, eating breakfast offers benefits like improved concentration, reduced risk of cardiovascular disease, and improved strength and endurance later in the morning. It is a no-brainer that eating breakfast is one habit that you should adopt if you haven't already.

For someone who is not used to eating breakfast, you will need to adopt some tricks.

For many years I was a breakfast-skipper myself. The only thing I used to consume in the morning was a glass of milk. In fact, I started eating breakfast regularly after I started losing weight, as I did not know any better.

There are a few considerations that will help you in acquiring the habit of eating breakfast.

One of the key requirements is that you take breakfast in the morning. If you're in the habit of getting up late in the morning and rushing to work, then you will find it much more difficult to eat breakfast in the morning. You need to set aside a chunk of time in the morning in order to eat breakfast. This can be only done if you wake up earlier than your usual waking up time. If you're a night owl, I can recommend the book *The Miracle Morning* by Hal Elrod. It teaches you how to wake up early, thus giving you enough time to eat breakfast.

Another reason that I was disinclined to take breakfast in morning was that I did not feel hungry enough to eat anything. This happens if there is only a short interval between when you wake and the time you eat breakfast. If you wake up earlier than you normally do not only to end up having time on hand for eating breakfast, but also you'll develop an appetite for eating breakfast. Another way to ensure your appetite for breakfast is to incorporate walking or exercise in the morning

So what should you eat in the morning?

You should be aware of a few important nutritional principles that make an ideal breakfast. As long as you adhere to them, you can literally have anything you like. There are three things to remember in this regard:

1. You should aim to meet 15-25% of your daily caloric intake from your breakfast. For example, if you determined from the nutrition table that you need 2,000 calories a day, your breakfast should have anywhere between 300-500 calories.

2. Breakfast should include high protein foods, such as eggs, lean meats or dairy products.

3. Along with protein, you should consume some complex carbohydrates with a high fiber content such as whole grains and fresh fruit. Avoid adding refined sugar to your cereal.

4. The ideal breakfast would be rounded off with some

fruits juice or low-fat dairy products that will provide you with calcium.

If you look at what you have been eating for breakfast, you might realize that you have been missing protein. It is the single most important constituent of a healthy breakfast that can help you to lose weight. Proteins eaten in the morning will keep you feeling full for most of the morning, thus preventing you from mid-morning snacking.

The Breakfast Eating Habit

If you are not used to eating breakfast regularly and want to lose weight, you will need to pick up the habit. Not only does breakfast come first in the day's meals, but is also first in terms of importance. Eating or omitting breakfast has the maximum influence on causing weight loss compared to lunch or dinner.

In order to eat breakfast in the morning regularly, you need three things, time, appetite and the food itself. Let me take you through each constituent separately and address how you can prepare for it.

There is no doubt that you need some extra time in the morning if you want to make breakfast into a habit. If you barely have enough time to get ready in the morning and get to work then you will find it very difficult logistically to take up this habit. You need a slot of at least 15 minutes in the morning in order to prepare and eat breakfast. The only way you can find this extra time is if you wake up a little earlier than you normally do. Set your alarm 15 minutes earlier than it is set currently, and it should do the job.

The next thing you need is to do some prep work in the kitchen the night before. Think of all possible steps that you need to undertake to prepare your breakfast, identify whatever can be done on the night before and then do it. Leave yourself the minimum possible amount of work for the morning.

You breakfast should be simple to prepare and it should be consistent. This solves a lot of problems including reducing the time required to prepare it in the morning and more importantly it becomes easier to adopt as a habit.

I usually have a bowl of oatmeal, some nuts, dried berries, milk and cottage cheese. This satisfies all the nutritional requirements and it's simple to prepare. Even on weekends when I might be having a fancier brunch, I still eat these foods first so that when I get to the fancy portion of the meal I do not end up gorging on it.

Portion Size

Most of us are food finishers. Think about it.

In childhood, we were trained to finish all the food that was put in front of us. This habit is so deeply ingrained that we continue to adhere to it long into adulthood.

Eating at a restaurant is a good way to understand this concept. We are being served ever increasing sizes of entrees in restaurants and yet on most occasions, we manage to finish whatever we order. It doesn't matter how much food comes on our plates, all of it usually ends up in our stomachs. Another example is packaged food, like snacks. Have you ever noticed that the packaging size of things like chips and cookies has been growing over the years? Yet, we eat them by the packet. This means that we are eating a constantly increasing quantity of these snacks, probably without even realizing it.

So how do you control portion size and thereby caloric intake?

There are several measures that you can take. The easiest to control are the packaged foods. Whenever you are buying something pre-packaged, go for the smallest available size. If you think you will not be happy with it, you can buy another one, but don't begin with a large size of anything. This can apply to many things like ice cream, chips, even beverages.

When it comes to your main meals, try not to fill up your plate at once. You should always see some empty space on your plate.

When eating outside of your home, try and share your entree. Another trick to limit portion size is to ask the server to pack half of the entree before it is even served. Trust me, you wouldn't even notice that you have been served only half an entree, now that they have become so big.

The idea is that you should become aware of portion sizes. Once you do, you can start figuring out how to control them.

Snacking

When someone says the word snacking, what is the first thing that comes to mind? Potato chips? Pretzels? Peanuts?

Traditionally, when we talk about snacking, we think of the time when we eat high energy density, dry, pre-packaged food like the one I mentioned above. This is only partly true.

The single most effective intervention that can prevent you from binging on high-caloric snacks occurs at the point of purchase. That's right, you have got to stop right at the origin. Start by looking at the nutrition labels carefully. A common folly that people make is to look at the calories per serving size. In an ideal world where you would eat only one serving, this information would be sufficient. However, you know better. Almost every time you buy a bag of chips, you end up eating much more than one serving. Probably, the whole bag. So instead of looking at the calories present in one serving, look at the number of calories contained in the entire pack. This will give you a better idea of how much it will cost calorie wise to you. For example, if you buy a bag of pretzels that contains 20 servings, with each serving of about 120 calories, you have in effect bought for yourself a bag worth 2,400 calories. You may exercise restraint and eat only one serving at a time. Still, over time you will end up consuming those 2,400 calories. The idea is, if you buy it, you will eat it. So, the best way to avoid these calories is to not stock up on them. Instead, go for low energy density snacks like butter-free popcorn. When you use the biological definition of snacks, then even fruits are considered snacks.

Distractions While Eating

Older times must have been simpler. Eating was a form of entertainment by itself. It still is to an extent but in a lot of homes, eating meals in front of the television is quite common. Studies have shown that children eat 167 extra calories for every hour of television they watch. Watching television while eating food can make you consume more through various means. The images of food being prepared and the advertisements about food can prompt you to eat more. At a more generic level, if you are watching TV while having your dinner, you don't realize how much you are actually eating. Being distracted by any means will lead you to consume more calories than you would if you are not doing anything else while eating. These activities include reading a book and even texting.

So, a simple thing to do is to switch off the television while eating or put away the newspaper for a while. This simple change can have a meaningful impact on your caloric intake.

Eating Reflexes

Pavlov was a Russian scientist who is known for his experiments on conditioned reflexes. He noticed that dogs salivated when they were served food. In his experiments, he would ring a bell whenever the dogs were served food. After this was repeated over a length of time, the dogs started associating the ringing of the bell with food. After a period of conditioning, the dogs would salivate just hearing the bell ring. This is what was known as conditioned reflex.

To an extent, our eating habits function like conditioned reflexes. Let me give an example here. At my workplace, we have a designated lunch hour from 1 PM to 2 PM. I am used to taking lunch every day at this time. I noticed that wherever I might be in the world, I started feeling hungry whenever the clock struck one in the afternoon. I am talking about real, stomach rumbling sort of hunger. The only explanation is that I have developed a conditioned reflect for lunch that is triggered by knowing it is 1 PM. So how do you harness this knowledge in your weight loss effort? Your job is to first identify if you have any conditioned reflexes regarding eating. Are there any particular times of the day or situations when you definitely eat? Those can be the potential occasions where you might have developed reflex eating habits. Examples of these situations are grabbing a cookie in the office when having a coffee or always reaching for a piece of chocolate after dinner. Look carefully into your day for such examples. Once you identify them, you can work on reducing their impact. You do this through preparation. In my case, having realized that I would get hunger pangs at 1 PM, I made sure to carry a healthy, nutritious lunch with me every day from home. I also made sure that I could eat it at around 1 PM, as often as possible. In this way whenever my conditioned reflex would strike, I had access to some healthy food.

Small Habits to Reduce Caloric Intake

Aside from the relatively bigger approaches that I have talked about earlier, there are some "micro" habits that you may consider that can help you in reducing your caloric intake. These habits are small by themselves but have a large impact on your diet.

Brush Your Teeth Right After Dinner

If you start following the earlier recommended habits, you would notice that there is a substantial time gap between dinner and bed time. Although this has a great beneficial effect on your caloric intake and sleep quality, it may leave you vulnerable in the period after dinner and the time you go to bed. There is a tendency for snacking during this time. To make things worse, usually you go for energy dense things like cookies and ice cream to satisfy yourself.

A habit that you may adopt is to brush your teeth right after dinner. This acts like a mental full stop to your brain, regarding food intake for the night. Once you have brushed your teeth, you will be much less likely to reach for that scoop of ice cream.

The key is to brush your teeth immediately after dinner so that you don't allow any time for night snacking.

Eating Out

Approximately one third of daily calorie consumption in the United States comes from away-from-home foods. This is a huge fraction. The principles which I have talked about previously apply to eating away from home also. However, these situations need some special attention.

When you eat out, you end up consuming almost twice as much energy compared to an average meal at home. Moreover, if you're eating fast food you will also consume more total fat, more added sugars, more sugar sweetened beverages, less fiber, less milk and fewer non-starchy vegetables. In effect, you do exactly opposite of what is required to lose weight.

Let us try and understand why this happens. There is a tendency to eat foods high in energy density when dining out, food that have a high fat content and contain fewer ingredients with high moisture content such as fruits and vegetables. There is also a tendency to eat larger portions. And lastly, there is more variety at restaurants. The more variety that you see, the more you are likely to overeat. Think of the last time you ate a buffet. Did you stuff yourself silly? I am sure of it.

By now you have understood that eating out presents multiple challenges to your weight loss efforts. Hence, you need to have a multi-pronged defense against this onslaught of calories. The first thing to remember is to not feel forced to do exactly as the restaurant tells you to do. The staff at a restaurant are trained to push you towards ordering more. Remember the documentary *Supersize Me*? Here's how you can avoid falling into this trap:

Look for words like steamed, broiled, baked, roasted or poached in the menu descriptions. They are likely to have lesser calories than anything that is fried.

- Choose a red sauce over a cream sauce.
- Try and select a thin soup or salad as a starter.
- Vegetarian meals are generally less calorie dense than non-vegetarian meals.
- Always try and select desserts which at least consist partially of fresh fruit.
- Control the size of your portion. Order a half portion, share your meal with a companion, or ask the server to pack half of your meal before it is served.

The important thing is to be aware of the pitfalls of eating out and apply at least one or a few of these strategies while doing so. I don't want you to end up eating a bowl of raw cabbage in a French restaurant! But at the same time, there is no need for you to consume double the amount of calories than you would have at home. Once you learn to strike a balance between the two extremes, you will enjoy your meals out and at the same time lessen their impact on your weight.

The 6 o'clock trap

Gary Keller, in his book *The One Thing*, talks about willpower. He says that willpower is like a tank of gas. We begin the day with a full tank of gas. As the day progresses, we summon our willpower as and when required. Tasks like implementing new behaviors, resisting temptation, suppressing impulses, and selecting long-term or short-term rewards all require willpower. So when we are faced with situations that require one of these actions on our behalf, some of our willpower for the day is used. Some tasks require more, and some less, but all of them keep emptying our willpower tank. So as the day comes to a close, our willpower is diminishing. When we reach home, tired and hungry, with little willpower left in the tank, our healthy food habits give way. In a sense, we don't have anything left to overcome our urge to eat. We end up eating whatever is brought in front of us. And this is the genesis of the 6 o'clock trap. Another way to look at this is that when we start our day, we find it easier to stick to our healthy food habits. And as the day progresses, so do the mistakes.

So the question is how to tackle it. Summoning willpower is certainly not the answer, as it is clear that willpower comes only in limited quantities and when we're talking about the 6 o'clock trap we are running on empty. So there is no point in telling you to simply overcome the urge eat unhealthy foods. It is not going to work, because you may not have any remaining willpower left to do so. The next best option is to create an alternative that is better for you. It is imperative that you plan for this situation in the morning. What you need is a choice of foods that you like that are voluminous in nature and yet are lower in caloric value as compared to some of the high-calorie prepackaged snacks that you would normally eat in the evening. Some examples are salad, egg white preparations, butter free popcorn, and even fruit salads. The key is that these food items should be ready to eat before you reach home. There cannot be any lag time between when you reach home and you accessing these foods.

Another method that I have found useful to escape this trap is to shift up my dinner time. So that the 6 o'clock time for snacks actually is my new dinner time. I know this may not be possible for many of you, but do consider it. Even if you cannot shift dinner as early as 6 o'clock, try to bring it closer to 6 o'clock as much is possible.

Food Finisher

Paul Siegel, a psychologist from the University of Alabama and one of the pioneers of food research, in 1957, found that people have a 'completion compulsion' or tendency to eat entire servings or units of food. If you are offered a cookie for example, irrespective of the size, you will tend to finish it, rather then leave a part on the plate. In most cultures it is considered bad manners to leave food on the plate. So a lot of times, even if you feel full, you will still go ahead and try to finish whatever is left. In many households the mothers will finish whatever their children have left on the plate. You can stop doing this. Put away your plate as soon as you feel full. The longer you linger over a half eaten plate, the more likely are you to nibble on the leftover morsels.

I know it sounds a little selfish. Yes, I understand that there are a lot of people in the world do not get two square meals a day and I am telling you to leave food on the plate. I'm sorry to say this is one habit you'll have to adopt. You can help the world in other ways, but this is something you need to do if you are trying to lose weight.

Summary

You might be feeling a little overwhelmed by all the information in this section. I have reduced it down to the following core principles and habits:

• Be aware of what and how much you eat. Don't eat anything mindlessly.

• Start working on the habit of eating a nutritionally comprehensive breakfast each morning.

• Focus on eating proteins and cutting down on fats.

• Eliminate or reduce added sugars in your food and drink

• Learn and apply the principles of lowering energy density of food

• Remember to enforce all these principles even when you are eating out

These habits are easy to adopt and are capable of helping you control your caloric intake to the level where you can easily manage your weight.

CHAPTER FIVE

Pedometer Use:
The Second Keystone Habit

"Physical fitness is not only one of the most important keys to a healthy body, it is the basis of dynamic and creative intellectual activity."

—John F. Kennedy

Physical activity is the second part of the weight loss equation. While daily self-weighing governs your caloric intake restriction, physical activity will be governed by the use of a pedometer.

Pedometer

"Measurement is the first step that leads to control and eventually to improvement. If you can't measure something, you can't understand it. If you can't understand it, you can't control it. If you can't control it, you can't improve it."

— H. James Harrington, performance improvement guru

The Trabant—Travi, as it was more popularly known—was a car produced in East Germany in the 1970s. Among its many quirks was the fact that it had no fuel gauge. Drivers had no idea how much fuel they were starting with or how much farther they could go. The driver had to stop the car, get out, pull up the hood, and insert a dipstick into the fuel tank just to get an idea of how much fuel remained. Sound outlandish? Hard to imagine?

Well, this kind of inconvenience is part of everyday life for those who are not using a pedometer. Without one, we are like the Travi, lacking a fuel gauge or an odometer. Without a pedometer, we have no idea how far we have walked in a day, nor do we know what we need to do to control our weight.

A pedometer is a small electronic device about the size of a AAA battery that you carry with you or wear like a wrist watch. It measures the number of steps you take, objectively capturing body movement and providing information on the total amount, intensity, duration, and frequency of physical activity.

In effect, it confers measurability and goal setting capabilities to an open-ended entity like physical activity.

What is Physical Activity?

If left to our own devices, many amongst us would skip physical exercise. For those and others, there is some good news. You don't have to exercise to lose weight. You read that right. You don't have to exercise to lose weight. Let me clarify this: In order to lose weight, what you do have to do instead is physical activity and not physical exercise.

But aren't the two, physical exercise and physical activity the same thing, you might ask.

They are not the same thing and therein lies one of the keys to weight management.

The distinction between the two entities was clarified as late as in 1985 by Caspersen and colleagues from the Center for Disease Control and Prevention. They defined physical activity as "any bodily movement produced by skeletal muscles that results in energy expenditure." The key phrase is "any bodily movement." Every time that you move your body during the day, for any reason, it counts as physical activity.

Think of all the occasions that require you to physically move: going to the bathroom, cooking, making your bed, answering the door... in fact, almost everything that you do when you are not sleeping involves physical activity. Caspersen goes on to clarify that exercise is a sub-category of physical activity. It is a type of physical activity that is planned, structured, repetitive, and intentional.

Whenever you perform an activity in a sustained, regimented manner, it counts as exercise. In my view, it is regimented nature of exercise that intimidates most of us. There is also a social element we fear.. For some, it conjures images of svelte women running in leggins on the road or beefed up men lifting heavy weights in the gym. The images themselves are so daunting that they are enough to put off anyone who is fat and who is thinking of doing something active about losing weight.

Samantha Thomas from Monash University in Australia, studied people living with obesity and their attempts to lose weight, their attitudes towards dieting, physical exercise and weight loss solutions and finally, why their weight loss attempts have failed. When these people were asked about exercising, there seemed to be even more barriers in their way than when they spoke about dieting. The majority of participants said that they found exercising difficult because of their weight, physical health problems, that they could not afford gym subscriptions, or personal trainers, did not have time to exercise, or felt uncomfortable or embarrassed about taking part in organized exercise. The researchers went deeper into their reasons for not exercising, and found that these included, "it is dark when I get home from work, so I can't go for a walk," "feeling fat," "too lazy," and "I can't be bothered." Participants stated that it was very difficult to exercise on their own, and wanted someone else to motivate them. "Give me a personal trainer that gets me out of bed every morning and makes me exercise, and yeah, I'd lose weight."

Thankfully, you don't have to depend on exercise to lose weight. Physical activity will suffice.

Physical activity is a very broad category in that sense and gives you a lot of flexibility in terms of timing and the actual process. You are not bound by any time, place or resource constraints in order to do physical activity.

If you share the same concerns or excuses as the people in the Australian study, it is time to let go of them. Understanding the concept of physical activity and its dissimilarity to exercise will be a game changer in your weight loss efforts.

The regimented nature of exercise does offer some advantages though. You can measure the exact amount of energy expended while doing exercise. You can know this by simply keeping a tab of the distance that you run or knowing the number of laps that you swim. This also allows you to set targets for yourself for the day that you could aim to fulfill while exercising. For example, setting a goal to jog for two miles or swim ten laps in the pool. The open-ended nature of physical activity makes it less quantifiable.

Until now.

The arrival of the pedometer has shifted the paradigm.

Advantages of a Pedometer

If I could summarize the benefits of a pedometer in one line, it would be this: a pedometer makes an open-ended entity like physical activity measurable. Pedometers can objectively measure most of the physical activity that one might undertake in a day, which is precisely what you need. And then it goes a step further. In contrast to a formal exercise regimen, which requires you to allocate chunks of time during your day to a workout, a pedometer allows you to log physical activity in increments of one step at a time. That is the biggest advantage of using a pedometer to monitor your physical activity—not a single step that you take is wasted, and everything is logged. This logging of each step converts it into a game, in which you compete with yourself.

Logging the number of individual steps you take is the most basic function of the device, but most models also measure the number of floors you climb as well as the number of active minutes and number of calories expended each day. The latest models also track your sleep patterns and heart rate. Most of the devices can be connected to a computer or smart phone through specialized software applications. They present easy-to-understand graphs detailing information about your activity on a daily, weekly, monthly, and even yearly basis.

When we drive a car, we receive continuous feedback from

the instrument cluster. We can view our speed, distance traveled, and remaining fuel. We are so used to this information that we often fail to realize its importance and take its availability for granted. Think about driving a car with no information panel. The pedometer is to your physical health what the information cluster is to your driving. It continually tracks your movements and gives continuous feedback about the distance you've covered. Furthermore, by setting goals for yourself, it will keep you motivated to work harder, longer.

A group of researchers from the Ataturk University in Turkey studied 84 obese women to assess the efficacy of the pedometer. These women were randomly divided into two groups. The intervention group was assigned a diet and exercise regimen and given pedometers. The control group was prescribed a similar diet and exercise regimen but without pedometers. Both groups were given a three-month follow-up plan. At the end of the study, the researchers found that women in both groups lost weight, but the women with pedometers lost an average of *nine pounds* more than those without pedometers. To further substantiate the pedometer's role in this weight loss, the researchers found that the women with pedometers walked an average of 1000 more steps per day than their pre-experiment numbers, which equates to an extra half mile per day and translates into about 70 extra calories burned per day. These accelerated results were achieved by simply wearing a pedometer.

Imagine boarding an elevator. You might instinctively reach for the control panel and press the button for the floor you want to reach. Now, for a moment, imagine that the elevator has no labels—no information about the floor you are on and no way to let you know how far down you have descended. It sounds ridiculous, but this is similar to trying to increase your activity level without using a pedometer. You have no objective idea about your baseline activity level and therefore no idea about the measured improvements you may be making. Setting a daily target also gives you something to aim for and subsequently something to achieve on a regular basis.

In a meta-analysis (a study of studies) that evaluated the role of pedometer use in nine weight loss experiments, participants increased their daily walking by a minimum of a mile per day just by using a pedometer. No diet modification was involved in any of these studies; just by wearing a pedometer, participants lost an average of a pound of weight every ten weeks. Although this result may not sound impressive, imagine how this would improve if the participants also made lifestyle changes.

In a study in the Journal of the Amercan Medical Association researchers collected results from 26 studies on pedometers and health. They found that using a pedometer led to an average increase of around 2,200 steps per day for each participant, or approximately one extra mile of walking. The researchers found that pedometers were effective in increasing activity levels only when the users set a target goal for themselves. They also found that users managed to decrease their blood pressure by four points after they started using the pedometers. This is one side effect that medical professionals would enjoy seeing! These studies demonstrate unequivocally that pedometers can be a key ally in helping anyone lose weight and improve personal health.

Not only do these devices quantify your activity, they also motivate you to do a little bit of extra work on an ongoing basis.

Using the Pedometer: The Keystone Habit

If I tell you to go build a house, it might sound insurmountable and vague. But if I tell you that the first step is digging a hole of a specific size and at a particular location, you are much more likely to succeed. Why? Now the task is small, finite, and measurable. Similarly, I am not just telling you to increase your physical activity. Instead, I am asking you to start wearing a pedometer every day. At this point you don't even have to think about the physical activity part, just focus on wearing the pedometer, every day.

Doing this is not hard to do. It adds only a couple of seconds to your daily routine and won't disturb what you are otherwise doing.

This fulfills the two criteria that turn a regular habit into a keystone habit. The change that it demands from you is very small and but once the change is made, it set into motion a chain of events. In this case, wearing a pedometer will inspire self-awareness about your level of physical activity. Later, it will inspire the activity itself.

Unlike exercising, I cannot think of any excuse for not wearing a pedometer.

Neither can you.

Pedometer Buying Guide

Before going out and buying a pedometer, it is helpful to understand the various features that are available. Then, depending on your preference, you can buy the appropriate model.

The pedometer market has exploded over the last couple of years. Since it will be a vital tool for you in you weight loss endeavor, I suggest that you buy the best one you can afford. If you need any help in justifying the cost to yourself or a significant other, remember that commercial weight loss programs are estimated to cost about $350 for every pound shed. Compared to those, the cost of a pedometer is chump change.

Essentially, there are two types of pedometers available. The most common one looks like a pen drive, and you either keep it in your pocket or clip it to your clothing. The advantage of this type of pedometer is that it is unobtrusive, so you don't make a show of having one. The primary disadvantage is that it is more likely to be lost without you noticing it immediately. The other type of pedometer is worn like a watch, around your wrist. An obvious advantage to this type is that since it is always visible, you are less likely to lose it. Since it is visible to everyone, however, some users may not like it.

You also have to decide if you want a model that comes with a display. I recommend that you buy this type. The main purpose of a pedometer is to give you continuous feedback about your daily activity level. You will be able to have this only if you can see your data on the display. In the models without the display, you have to open the connected app on you phone to check the number of steps taken. It adds an additional step to the whole thing, one that you can avoid if you have a pedometer with its own display.

You can also purchase models that continuously measure your heart rate. If you are like me and really enjoy gadgets, you might consider buying this type of pedometer. I don't see any harm in receiving extra information about my activity and body, since I am going to be wearing a pedometer anyway.

Recommended Models of Pedometers

- Fitbit One: This is a pen-drive type of pedometer. It comes with a display and has a very good app for your smart phone. You can clip it to your clothing or keep it in your pocket. The battery life is quite good, as you need to charge it only once every ten days.

- Fitbit Charge HR: This pedometer is worn on your wrist, like a watch. Besides functioning as a pedometer, it also measures your heart rate by your wrist pulse. It is also waterproof, and you can even wear it while sleeping. I find that compliance with the wrist-worn models is better than those with clip-on models.

- Fitbit Surge: This pedometer has all the capabilities of the Charge HR model with the addition of GPS. If you like to walk or run outdoors, it may be useful for you. However, it is much bulkier than the above models, hence may not be suitable for all day wear.

If I had to recommend one model at present, it would be the Fitbit Charge HR.

Adopting The Keystone Habit

Your first task is to get used to wearing a pedometer every day and at all times.

Although it sounds like a small task, I find that adopting even this habit requires effort.

You are looking at doing two things here. One is getting used to wearing the pedometer every day. The second is doing it right in the morning, before you start moving around. In order to train yourself to do this, you need to tie this new habit to an old habit that you already might have.

Look at your daily morning routine in minute detail to find such a pre-existing habit. If you take a certain medication in the morning, then you could start keeping the pedometer next to that bottle of medicine. Whenever you reach for your medication each morning, you will automatically see the pedometer and wear it. If you wear contact lenses, you are already used to removing them right before going to bed and putting them in the first thing each morning. So, you could consider keeping the pedometer next to your contact lens case. Almost everyone uses a smart phone these days, and it must be charged regularly. You could keep your pedometer next to your smart phone or even on top of it.

Pick one of these habits, and tie the pedometer to it. In this way, the existing habit will lead you to develop another habit— in this case, wearing the pedometer every day beginning each morning. And, once you develop this keystone habit, many new habits will be triggered that will help you significantly increase the extent of your daily physical activities. Remember, you will need to wear it every day for the rest of your life.

It may sound intimidating here, me talking about wearing a gadget for a lifetime. However, you will soon realize that the pedometer trains you over a period of time in becoming an expert at judging your level of daily physical activity. And as this happens, you will slowly become less and less dependent on the pedometer to keep your physical activity up to the required level.

Initially, you may frequently look at your step count. You may do this many times a day when you are just starting out, which is very normal and expected. Over time you will start to develop a sense of correlation between your routine and the number of steps it leads to. Slowly, you will need to refer to the pedometer less and less to know the number of steps you have taken. Your body and brain will develop their own sense of the amount of physical activity that you undertake. In a sense, the brain will develop its own pedometer. Yes, you still will need to wear an actual pedometer, but your dependence on it to judge your level of physical activity will decline to a degree where you might just look at it once a day.

For my part, I have been wearing a pedometer for almost eight years now. Now that is has become an "old" habit for me, I don't even think about it. It just happens automatically. Wearing a pedometer is like wearing a wrist watch. You wear a wrist watch everyday. How many times do you need to look at it? Not much, I am guessing. Yet, if there is a day when for some reason you forget to wear your watch, that is the day you miss it. Same is true of the pedometer. I have maintained a daily count of more than 10,000 steps for many years, but I hardly need to look at my pedometer during the day, much like my wrist watch. (OK, I am fond of watches and don't like to use my smartphone for knowing the time, so maybe I am a little old-fashioned!) I have adapted myself to the point where I know exactly how many steps are the result of a particular action.

You should wear the pedometer as soon as you wake up and keep it on at all times. This is important because you want to account for every step. Unless you wear it all the time every day, you will not know accurately how much you have walked that day. And, unless you have an accurate step count, any kind of competition you are trying to have with yourself will be invalid. The idea is to capture every step that you take. Only then does the pedometer become useful. A sign that it has really become second nature is when you feel miserable if you forget to wear it. That is a sure indicator that it is becoming a habit.

Establish A Baseline Activity Level

Before you start using the pedometer to increase your activity level, you need to establish your own baseline level of daily activity.

These days there is a magic figure of "10,000" daily steps being bandied around, as if it were a panacea for all things bad with your health, including being a cure for obesity. This advice is as accurate as saying that everyone should weigh 130 pounds. 130 pounds may be an ideal weight for some people of a particular height, but it cannot be a target weight for the entire population. Similarly, you need to establish your own target for the number of steps you take each day. And this number will change over time, as you make progress.

The first step in getting to know your daily target is to determine where you currently stand in terms of the number of steps that you already take.

You will need a weeks' time to calculate your baseline activity level. The best time to start doing this is the weekend, more precisely Sunday. By starting the measurement on a Sunday and ending it on the subsequent Saturday, you will be able to capture the variations in the activity level that are expected to occur during different days of the week.

Start wearing the pedometer daily, beginning Sunday morning, at all times. Use the tricks that I have described before to make sure that you put it on in the morning and keep it on you at all times. You should ensure that as far as possible, you stick to doing what you normally do during these days. I know that you are highly motivated to raise your activity level, but control your urge to increase your activity during this week. You don't want to have a falsely elevated baseline level as this will make it very difficult for you to increase it from there.

You should conduct this measurement during a week that mirrors your normal week in terms of your daily routine. If you have something unusual planned in the week like extended travel, consider deferring this measurement. We are looking to capture a snapshot of what your regular week looks like in terms of physical activity.

The average number of baseline steps taken by individuals varies widely depending on the country or even the state in which the individual lives. On an average, American adults take approximately 6,500 steps per day. Japanese people are a little ahead in this regard and walk almost 7,200 steps per day. Europeans walk even more than the Americans or the Japanese. Amongst the Europeans, Belgian and Swiss adults come out on top, each managing to walk almost 10,000 steps per day. The Amish however are the undisputed champions in the steps game. On an average, an Amish adult accumulates a massive 18,000 steps every day, probably due to the fact that they don't use automobiles.

The average national figures will give you a rough idea of where you stand at the moment vis a vis others in the step count ladder.

What is most important is that within a week, you will establish a baseline of your own level of physical activity. This would serve as a foundation for making progress on the physical activity front.

Set a Daily Target for Number of Steps

Now that you have established a baseline figure of your daily physical activity, the next step is to set a daily target for yourself.

Pedometer use by itself has moderate benefits in terms of increasing physical activity. The real benefit of using a pedometer is to set daily step count goals for yourself. In fact, it has been seen that people who create a daily step count goal manage to significantly increase their physical activity.

A meta-analysis was conducted to evaluate the role of setting goals while using pedometers. It found that participants in studies that did not include a step goal showed no significant improvement in physical activity with pedometer use. On the other hand, participants in studies that incorporated specific goals increased their daily physical activity by almost 2,000 steps.

There are a few things to consider here.

The target you set for yourself should be realistic. There is no point in setting a goal of 10,000 steps per day when your current baseline level is only 4,000 steps. You will find it very difficult to achieve your goal on most days, and failure to do so will lead to frustration.

So, how do you set a target? Let us figure this out backwards.

Consider this fact: When walking at a moderately brisk pace, the average adult takes about 100 steps per minute, which is about 1,500 steps per 15 minutes of walking. Based on this fact, adding 1,500 steps per day is a realistic addition to your baseline, whatever it might be at present. And the 15 minutes required to do so is not much time required either. So, aim for an additional 1,500 steps over your baseline level when you begin. Assuming you started with an average of 4,000 steps, your target now becomes 5,500 steps per day. You can do the simple arithmetic to calculate your individual daily target. Just add 1,500 steps to your baseline number.

Now that you have a daily target, you must aim to achieve it. Take each day one by one. Your aim should be to cross the daily step target every single day.

If you try and achieve your daily target every day, you will likely overshoot. This is because you don't stop moving for the day after having reached your target. A runner who is trying to finish a 5k run does not stop dead in his tracks once he reaches the finish line; he goes on for some distance. Similarly, you will keep on moving even after you reach your goal. So, depending on the time of the day that you reach your target, you are sure to pile on extra steps over your goal. This is why it is even more important to achieve your step goal on a daily basis.

Achieving Your Daily Steps Target

"The greatest danger for most of us is not that our aim is too high and miss it, but that our aim is too low and we reach it."

—Michelangelo

"Give me a stock clerk with a goal and I'll give you a man who will make history. Give me a man with no goals and I'll give you a stock clerk."

—J.C. Penney, American businessman and entrepreneur, founder of the J. C. Penney stores

Having set a daily target of the number of steps you wish to take, you now have a goal—one that is finite, measurable, and visible from where you stand today. These are important criteria that determine the probability of hitting your target. To achieve your daily goal, think of the day ahead, not the week or the month. Take just one day at a time.

As far as the daily step target is concerned, you have to invest one minute of your time in the morning to plan how you are going to achieve the step target. You have to consider things like your schedule for the day. On some days, you will have back-to-back meetings, on some you will be traveling, and on others you will need to attend an unavoidable event.

If it is a standard day, then you know exactly what you are going to be doing and when you are going to be doing it. You also know that these activities will lead you to getting to your baseline level of steps. Your job now is to simply see where and how you can squeeze in the extra 1,500 steps required to reach the daily target. If you walk at a brisk pace, then you need just 15 minutes to gather the extra 1,500 steps. You can accumulate them either in one go or in parts. Try parking your vehicle a little farther away than usual. To reach your office, your class, or wherever you are supposed to be, try taking the stairs. Then, during the day, get up and take a short walk around your work-place. You might be thinking that you are already aware of these things, but the important difference is that now you are logging all these efforts. Everything counts. Even if you stand up while talking on the phone or when you get up to go to the bathroom, your steps are logged. And each step takes you closer to your new target. The target now is not to lose 50 kilos; the target is to add 1,500 steps per day. That is the difference.

If it is not a typical day for you because you are either travelling or doing something that you normally don't do, you have a challenge ahead. Now you don't have to plan just for the additional 1,500 steps; you also have to think about first getting to your baseline number of steps. The easiest way to accomplish this is to go for a walk in the morning. You can do this outdoors or on a treadmill. I definitely try to do this on days when I am not sure about my routine. I hop onto my treadmill and try and add my baseline number of steps to my count. I am then mentally free for the rest of the day. I continue adding steps whenever I can, but I am at peace that I will not be coming back to my home in the evening with a backlog of 5,000 steps. That is crushing for my spirit.

Sometimes morning walks may not always be an option for some reason. If this is the case, I suggest that you become more vigilant and proactive during the day in regards to your step count. It is on these days that the pedometer has the maximum use. First, look at your step count more frequently through the day. Divide the day into three equal parts. The first part comes before lunch, the second between lunch and arriving back home, and the third between the time you reach home and bedtime. You have now divided your daily steps goal into three equal but smaller targets. Try to hit them individually. If your daily target is 9,000 steps, try to reach 3,000 before lunch, 6,000 by the time you return home, and any remaining before bedtime. If you follow this practice, you will not have a big backlog to cover at any point of the day. Try and squeeze in short bursts of steps whenever you see an opportunity. You don't need a running track to do it. Any time you see a hallway or an open space, try and get in some steps. Over time, as you encounter different scenarios, it will become less and less tedious.

Clinical studies have shown that using pedometers has many benefits. Participants decreased their BMI by .38 from their baseline number. They decreased their systolic blood pressure by 3.8mm Hg. Do not underestimate the importance of a 4mm BP reduction. Reducing systolic blood pressure by just 2mm is associated with a 10% reduction in stroke mortality and a 7% reduction in mortality from vascular causes in middle-aged populations. Accordingly, you would have significant health advantages.

Walking: The Only Exercise that you Need

"Walking is the best possible exercise. Habituate yourself to walk very far."
—Thomas Jefferson

President Jefferson was able to figure this out long ago, and he didn't have the benefit of having today's research at his disposal.

Walking is the most natural of all forms of physical exercise. Yes, exercise. I have purposely used the term physical exercise and not physical activity to describe walking. It may not seem like it, but walking, even at a leisurely pace, is considered to be a perfectly acceptable form of physical exercise.

When I set out to lose weight myself, I was under the impression, like many of you might be, that an activity doesn't count as exercise unless it leaves you out of breath or sweating. Anything less intense than that, I thought, is no good for weight loss. As someone who had been living a sedentary lifestyle almost all of my adult life, I knew I was miles away from any form of exercise. But then I learned the transformational effect that walking could have. And boy, did that change me.

I have a pop quiz for you. Which of the following activities do you think will burn more calories: running at full steam for one kilometer or walking the same distance?

If you answered that both are equal, then your understanding about the relationship between exercise and calories is on target. However, if you thought that running the same distance would result in a greater calorie burn, read on. You are in for a surprise.

The factor that determines the calories that a person spends performing an activity such as walking or running is the final distance covered and not the speed at which it is covered. So you may run, walk or even crawl to make your way across a kilometer, the calories that you spend covering that distance will essentially be the same, irrespective of your speed. This fact is difficult to digest at first. It seems to go against common sense. Remember the last time you were in park with a jogging track? You must have seen some people who were running on the track and some who were just walking. It might be difficult to believe that both would end up burning an equal number of calories, provided they covered the same distance.

To a casual observer, running and walking appear to be similar to each other, the only difference being the speed. This observation is incorrect. Running is not a faster version of walking. Both are very different activities in terms of the effort they require from the human body and also their relative impact on the body. Let me explain. When you are walking, one of you feet is always on the ground. However fast you may walk, only one foot comes off the ground at a time, while the other stays grounded. In contrast, when you start running, both your feet come off the ground together with each stride.

Have you ever seen the competitors in the Olympic event of fast walking? With their top speed touching almost 15 kilometres an hour, they give the impression that they are actually running and not walking. However it may appear to us, the truth is that they are walking. One of the things that can get them disqualified is lifting both feet off the ground, which is defined as running.

So why is this thing of one foot or both feet important for you? If you start running, both your feet come off the ground for a fraction of second before the foot that is ahead lands on the surface below. At that point of contact, when it lands, all your body weight falls on that foot. The shock wave that arises from that landing goes through the foot all the way up your leg, through your knee, to your spine. Can you feel the crunch already? If you are walking, none of this happens, as one of your feet is always grounded. The intensity of the impact depends on how much the person weighs. The higher one's weight, the higher the impact.

This is not to discourage you from taking up running in the future. But for the time that you are overweight, it is better that you stick to walking. The ill effects of running while being overweight don't end here. As an overweight person, your ability to balance your body is lesser than that of a person of normal weight. So you are more likely to fall and injure yourself when attempting to run. Also, as running expends energy at a higher rate than walking, you will run out of steam much earlier than you would while walking. This can be a big demotivating factor.

So, when you are in the initial phase of the weight loss process, it is better to concentrate on walking and stay away from the urge to run. Of course, as you lose weight and gain stamina, you can graduate to running. No wonder Jefferson has been considered one of the wisest people to have roamed the earth. He didn't need all these explanations to determine that walking is the best possible exercise.

Making Walking a Habit

"Typically, people who exercise, start eating better and becoming more productive at work. They smoke less and show more patience with colleagues and family. They use their credit cards less frequently and say they feel less stressed. Exercise is a keystone habit that triggers widespread change."

—Charles Duhigg, *The Power of Habit: Why We Do What We Do in Life and Business*

I hope that by this time you are sufficiently motivated to take up walking as form of exercise. If so, you have just completed the initiation phase of adopting this as a new habit.

The next step is to create the context or the situation that will prompt you to go for a walk automatically, everyday. To accomplish this, you need to mentally plan to go for a walk a day prior. You need to think about the most suitable time (morning/afternoon/evening) and place (outdoors/gym). In essence, you are scheduling an appointment for walking. You will see that this simple step will set into motion the chain of small steps that will enable you to go out the next day.

Our minds are quite fickle. They are always looking for excuses to avoid doing something that we are not used to doing or do not want to do. Exercise is one such example. One way to prevent this is to anticipate everything that you might need for your walk, and prepare in advance accordingly. So, lay out your exercise clothes, socks, and sports shoes the night before. Place these things where they are sure to catch your attention. If you plan on using things like a water bottle, heart rate monitor, or earphones, place them alongside your walking clothes. You shouldn't be looking for anything to take along at the last moment.

Once these physical objects are in place, you should state your intention out loud. "I have to go for a walk tomorrow morning at 7 A.M., no matter what," for instance. Of, course you can fill in your own time. Do this consciously, and set up an appointment with yourself. You will not believe how much this small act will help.

There are a couple of other small tricks that I used to get myself to go for walks regularly. When I was doing it in the evenings, I used to lay out my gear before I went to work in the morning. As soon as I returned home, I would change into my walking gear, shoes included. Only then would I proceed to eat or drink something. If I look back, I realize that this thing helped me in two ways. One, the change of clothes primed my brain for the fact that I would be soon going out for a walk, discouraging me from loading myself with the sort of energy dense snacks that I would previously eat. Second, it didn't allow me any leeway to get lazy and somehow miss my walk. Once you have changed into walking clothes and even more importantly, are wearing walking shoes, there is no turning back.

Once you get into these habits, they start to become automatic in nature.

Inside or Outside?

You can choose to walk on a treadmill or you can choose to walk outdoors. Both have advantages and disadvantages. Let me take you through them briefly.

Walking on a treadmill frees you from the vagaries of nature. If you live in a place that has a very harsh climate, you may not be able to go outdoors every day. There is no such problem if you walk on a treadmill. If you have a treadmill at home, you can be very flexible in the timing of your walking routine and work it into your daily schedule. This is especially true if you keep long hours at work, as you don't even have to step out of your home to go to a gym. Having a treadmill at home is also useful on days when you get home late and are falling short of your daily steps target and don't have the energy to go back outside. Instead, you can hop on to your treadmill, finish off the daily step goal, and do no more. Just making it to my daily step target on such days always gave me a great sense of achievement. I have done it more than a couple of times. Although, don't walk so late too often or else it will become a habit, one that you don't want to acquire!

If you decide to walk outdoors you have two options. You can either walk on along a trail or along the road. Walking on the road has the advantage of enabling your walk to begin the minute you step out of your house. Walking in a park or on a trail allows you to be in midst of nature, enjoying the chirping of birds, the smell of flowers, the sight of lush green trees, the fresh air. Nothing can beat the feeling. Also, you don't have to be on the lookout for oncoming traffic, as you have to do while walking on the road.

You don't have to choose one. I alternate between both options. On most days, I try to go to a nearby park for my walk, time and weather permitting. I use the treadmill in my home as a backup whenever I find that I am unable to go the park. The system is foolproof.

Going the Distance Outdoors

Walking outdoors can be a very pleasurable activity. No wonder it is the most common form of exercise in the United States, with 30% of the population walking regularly.

If you think about it, walking is the most natural physical movement that you can do. That is why people seem to love it. And if you do it outdoors, the pleasure is amplified.

I found that the single biggest advantage of walking outdoors is that you can cover long distances without boredom setting in.

When I had just started going for walks, I would find it intimidating in the beginning, especially if I thought about the distance I had to cover. In my case I was walking two laps around a two-kilometer track. In order to reduce my trepidation, I would focus on completing the half of the first round and forget about the total distance to be covered. By doing this, I had effectively reduced my first target from 4 kilometres to 1 kilometre and this made things much easier. Once I completed the first half of the lap, I told myself that I had completed one-fourth of the total distance to be covered. Then, keeping my focus on the next half, I would similarly finish it with ease. And once the first lap was over, I would get a great boost that the remaining distance was less than half of the total to be covered. You will see it for yourself, that once you cross the halfway mark, you do get a big mental boost and things get much easier from there. And with each meter of the second lap that I walked, the percentage of the remaining distance would diminish very fast. You can use this method to conquer any fear that you might have when just starting going for walks. Divide the distance that you plan to cover into small chunks and concentrate on each chunk individually.

You can keep yourself entertained by listening to either music or things like podcasts or even audio books while walking. Since walking can take a significant amount of my time, I now prefer to listen to podcasts rather than music in order to maximize the use of my time. Since you are walking, you can comprehend whatever is being said in the podcasts, something that is not easy to do if you are running.

Walking on a Treadmill

I have a treadmill at my home. I use it as a backup for those days when I am unable to go outdoors for a walk. This could be due to bad weather or for lack of time. Either way, just the knowledge that I have a treadmill to fall back upon gives me great peace of mind.

Walking on a treadmill can be a trifle boring in the beginning, but I've devised a few tricks to get over this apparent shortcoming.

Buying A Treadmill

I suggest you consider buying a treadmill if you can afford it and have the space in your house. You can take my word that it will be one of the best investments you ever make.

Over the years I have guided many friends on their treadmill purchases. Having used one for many years now, I have really simplified my advise on this aspect. There are only three things that will matter to you in a treadmill if you going to be using it for walking for weight loss. These are:

-Buy the widest treadmill that you can afford and have space for. The bigger the treadmill, the more conducive it will be for walking naturally. You should be looking for the widest belt possible, as I have seen that a narrow belt is the one of the biggest impediments to regular use of a treadmill. You should look for a width of 20 inches or more. Anything less than 18 inches wide is quite uncomfortable to use on a regular basis.

-The only add-on feature that I have found to be of a practical use is the ability to electronically change the incline of the walking surface. Raising the incline can have a dramatic effect on the calories burnt while walking.

It is equally important to know what features should not influence your purchase. There are two things that treadmill manufactures often tout as their unique selling proposition but really are quite useless in my opinion. The first is the added electronics like a television screen, mp3 player or even a small fan. Most of them are gimmicky and are of much lower quality than you can find if you were to buy them individually. With technology becoming better and cheaper by the day, there is no sense getting stuck with an outdated speaker or a small LCD screen fixed to your treadmill. And because these things are of such low quality, they go kaput in no time. Lastly, the manufacturers charge a huge markup on them.

The other thing I have found to be of little use is the built-in exercise programs. If you are going to be buying a treadmill for walking purposes only, you won't have much use for them. And again, the manufacturers seem to incorporate these features only to inflate the price. They are nothing but various permutations and combination of the treadmill speed and incline. On most occasions you just end up using the default setting.

However, there is one feature that you may look at favorably, this being the wireless heart rate monitoring. Most mid-level treadmills now come with a contact based heart rate monitor that measures your heart rate when you grab the handrails. It is better to invest in a machine with a wireless heart rate monitor, as it can give you a continuous, real time display of your heart rate without disrupting your natural walking rhythm. They don't require you to hold on to anything while you are walking, although you will need to wear a chest belt while. Real time heart rate feedback is a really cool feature and can be very useful in not only keeping you engaged while on the treadmill but can also guide you about the intensity of your workout.

Avoiding Boredom While on the Treadmill

Let's be frank. Walking on the treadmill can be boring, especially in the initial phases. That is why it is essential that you prepare some form of entertainment for yourself in advance.

In my own initial days of treadmill walking, I placed an iPad on a couple of hooks fixed on the console of the treadmill, which

I used to watch recorded episodes of my favorite television shows. One advantage of watching TV shows over watching movies is that they typically run for a standard duration of time. So on most occasions I ended up walking longer just to finish an episode. Movies, on the other hand, are long enough that they probably won't stretch your treadmill time.

The other, more traditional option is to listen to audio while walking. You may choose to listen to music. An alternate option is to listen to podcasts, which I find to be more engaging. Audio books are another option, and many of them are free.

Going the Distance

When you begin walking on the treadmill, you might feel unnerved by the distance you plan to cover.

Say you plan to walk for 4 miles. When your display indicates that the distance covered is only 0.5 miles, you have a reason to feel scared. The distance remaining looks daunting and you might feel that it is actually impossible to finish. Try this mental trick: Don't even think about your ultimate goal of 4 miles; concentrate on reaching the 1 mile mark. Once you reach that mark (this should take about 15 minutes at a normal walking pace for most), tell yourself that you have already finished one-fourth of the job. Set your next mental goal at 2 miles. Once you reach that (another 15 minutes), your mind will tell you half the distance is covered. From that point on, you can tell yourself that the distance remaining is less than whatever you have already walked. After that, it really becomes easy as you think of the remaining distance as a small percentage of the distance already covered. You will find that this method will really help you manage the task.

Pitfalls of the Treadmill

When you are just starting to walk on a treadmill, you may feel a sense of imbalance. To counter this you tend to hold on to to the rails. No problem in that. But do not continue to do this all the time. Not only does it impede your normal range of motion, but it also decreases the effort you're expending.

If you set the speed a little too high, then you will end up taking very long strides. If your stride length becomes much longer than your normal stride length, it will make things uncomfortable and you will max out quite early. So, aim to keep the speed at such a level that you don't need to take very long strides. Rather, increase the speed of walking than trying to take elongated strides.

Whenever you need to get off the treadmill, slow it down gradually. Don't jump off a moving treadmill. Not only is sudden stoppage of movement bad for the heart, but it also might cause you to fall.

Time To Up Your Target

Once you start hitting your daily step target on a consistent basis, it is time to move to the next level. A word of caution here: don't overextend yourself. If you reach your new target for a only a few days in succession and start thinking, "Ok, now that I have been doing 6,500 steps per day for a week, I think I should move up to 8,000 next week," think again.

Remember that you had a baseline number of steps when you started this journey. You have taken a lifetime to establish this baseline number. Even if you have managed to hit your targets for a couple of days, you body's "memory" is still comfortable with your original baseline. Before you move to the next level, you must make sure that you have become comfortable with your first target number of steps. The idea is that it should have become a new baseline. Once it is, you can safely build the next level on top of it.

There is an objective parameter to know when to raise your target. Research has shown that it takes an average of 66 days to establish a new habit—about two months. Once you start a new activity in your life, you have to make every effort to do it consecutively for 66 days before it becomes a habit. Once it does, that activity will happen with little conscious effort on your part. Now you know when your new target should become your new baseline. If you achieve your steps target consistently for 66 days (minus one or two), you have your new baseline.

If you maintain this goal after 66 days of having set a new target, you have earned yourself the right to set another even higher target. How much should the next increase be? Another 1,500 steps? Or maybe 2,000? No, that would be a bad idea. Have you seen a picture of the Egyptian pyramids? They have been around for more than 5,000 years. Among other factors accounting for their longevity is that they have a tapered structure. As you look upward, the number of stones per level decreases, which increases their stability and hence their longevity. I suggest you take the same approach with your daily steps target. If you successfully increase your target by 1,500 steps, the next increase should not be more that two-thirds that number. In this case, the new target would be 1,000 steps over your last target. The next increase should then be two-thirds of 1,000—approximately 650 steps—and so on until you reach a point where your increase is about 250. That is a level you don't pare down. Once you reach a level when your next increment becomes 250 steps, you can stop using this percentage method and use a standard increment of 250 steps. Remember that you are building a pyramid of your own. You want it to last a lifetime, so it has to be extremely stable. Each successive increase will be a little harder and a little more difficult to maintain than the last increase. Reducing each successive increase in the number of daily steps will make it more likely that you reach your goals.

A Few More Fitbit Features

It is very obvious that if you favor the stairs over the elevator, you will burn some extra calories. Pedometers can help here too. Most pedometers count the number of floors that you climb during the day by individually counting the number of stairs climbed. In fact, you can set a floor goal on the pedometer's phone app.

A logical question that may occur to you is whether stair-climbing is worth the effort. There are multiple benefits of climbing stairs that I can cite here. Climbing stairs is considered to be a "vigorous" form of exercise. A minute of stair-climbing will burn more calories than a minute of jogging. It saves time too. If you walk up five floors or less, then you are likely getting to your destination faster by taking the stairs than by taking the elevator. Climbing each floor burns about 1.5 calories, so aiming to climb at least ten floors a day will add up 15 calories a day. Since it is a time neutral activity, I consider it a complete bonus.

The floors climbed feature on your pedometer can help you maximize the caloric burn from climbing stairs. When you set targets for this feature, use the same principles that you used for setting goals for the number of steps you want to take per day. First determine a baseline level of the number of floors you climb on average from the data of your baseline week. Then add about 25% to this number. If you climbed an average of eight floors per day in your baseline week, add two floors.

Using the Summaries

An important way the pedometer provides positive feedback is through weekly and monthly summaries, which help you understand how consistent your activity has been in a particular week or month. If you find that your weekly or monthly averages are above your goal, then you have the satisfaction of knowing you are on the right track. You should keep reviewing your weekly and monthly stats regularly in addition to the daily numbers on the pedometer.

Using the Group Feature

The Fitbit app has a nifty feature that allows you to add people on your contact list to your Fitbit app account. In this way, you are in continuous competition with these contacts, which adds that little bit of extra motivation. After I had been using my pedometer for a long time, one by one all of my immediate family members took up Fitbit. Now I can see each one's step count on my app. I stay on top of this list most of the time, and I know this motivates the others to keep up.

Practical Tips about Using the Pedometer

The older models of pedometers that I used (Omron) came with replaceable batteries, much like those you find in a quartz wrist watch. These ran for months on end. My current model (Fitbit Charge HR) has a rechargeable battery. Since it also tracks my heart rate at all times, the device consumes a lot of power, and the battery runs for five to six days at most.

I have learned to keep an eye on the battery level. The paired Fitbit app on my phone does a good job of informing me when it is critically low. The best practice is to charge it whenever you get an opportunity to do so and not wait for the battery level to fall to a critically low level. This will ensure that you never end up walking around with a discharged pedometer! See, once you become used to tracking your steps on a daily basis, you will feel very frustrated if one day you find that your steps are not being logged just because you've been careless about the battery.

Pedometers can hold a limited amount of data. If they are set up by the manufacturers to hold data pertaining to the last week and month and keep deleting older data, make sure you keep it synchronized with your app. Once the data is transferred to the app, it becomes permanent, and you don't have to fear losing it. Current models of Fitbit are Bluetooth-enabled. Once you pair your phone with the pedometer, it automatically synchronizes the data across the pedometer and the app on the phone. So, with this feature it is no longer a chore to keep the data backed up.

Key Points to Remember

- A pedometer is to a person what a fuel gauge is to a car
- A pedometer will work only if you remember to wear it at all times
- Start with establishing a true baseline level of your physical activity
- Set a steps-per-day goal for yourself (+1500 steps over your current daily step level), and make sure you reach it every day
- Review your steps goal every month and make incremental additions to it after you have achieved your previous targets for two months at a stretch.

Regular pedometer use will add a mile of walking to your activity level each day

CHAPTER SIX

Traps: How To Escape Them

"Man is the only kind of vermin who sets his own trap, baits it, then steps in it."

—John Steinbeck, 1962 Nobel Prize winner for literature

You encounter traps on any road that you will travel on in life. The road to weight loss is no different. As you embark upon the journey towards weight loss you will come across traps that will pull you back. Your job is to avoid them.

The best way to avoid any trap is to be aware of it, and the best way to minimize the potential damage is to have a solid strategy in place for dealing with it beforehand.

Buffet Meals

There is something about free meals, even among the rich, that unleashes our desire to overeat. Buffet meals can derail the diet plans of even the most disciplined person. There are a few tricks that you can employ to escape the large dietary upheaval that can be brought about by a single buffet meal.

The single best defense is to avoid attending buffet meals altogether. It is easier than you think. List the last five buffet-type of meals that you went to. I'm sure if you do an objective cost-befit analysis, you could have avoided at least two or three of them without much problem. The price of a buffet meal will always be very attractive. It is designed that way. Don't fall into the trap. Always go for the à la carte option, if given one.

When your hand is forced and you have to pick up a plate at a buffet meal, use the energy density and pre-loading concepts that were covered in detail in the chapter on food.

Begin with a survey of the entire spread before you even pick up a plate. Then, start with a thin soup. Try to load up on salads before moving on to the main entrees. Having served yourself, try to be seated at a table that is the farthest away from the food table. Pre-loading with low energy density meals will greatly reduce the amount of high-calorie foods that you will consume later on. While serving yourself, try and put protein preferentially on your plate. The idea is that if you are going to be eating, let the calories come from proteins as much as possible. Eating proteins will make you full much sooner than carbs or fats. When eating, remember to consciously think about the point at which you stop feeling hungry. Try and stop eating at that point and get your plate cleared as soon as possible. Finally, be careful of the dessert menu. Typically these are quite extensive. Do enjoy it, but use portion control strategies to limit the caloric intake. Consider helping yourself to some fruit if available. That can reduce the caloric load brought upon by the dessert menu.

One final word: do not miss your weigh-in on the day after a buffet meal. You will most likely see a big jump in your weight, which will help to keep you in check the next time a buffet is in the offing.

Overnight Drop in Weight

Once in a while you may notice that your weight has dropped sharply, perhaps by as much as a couple of pounds over your previous day's weight. If you have been carefully reading this book, you can decipher on your own that this dramatic weight reduction cannot be attributed to the loss of solid mass in your body. You would need to shed 7,000 calories in order to lose two pounds of weight. That amount of caloric loss is unlikely to happen in a day.

How do you explain this sudden drop? Most of it is due to loss of water, not of body mass. The water loss itself mostly occurs as a result of missing a meal or two the previous day. When you rehydrate and eat your regular meals the next day, this sharp drop in weight reverses itself. That is why it is important to remember that this is a spurious finding. If you ever experience such a situation, keep these facts in mind and don't use it as an excuse to eat excessively.

Guilty Friends and Family

One thing about weight loss is that everyone wants to experience it themselves, but few are happy to see others achieve it. This is especially true if the person in question has failed at it. I've seen this happen a lot. If you think it sounds mean, recall the last time you saw one of your friends who had lost a significant amount of weight. How did you feel? More specifically, how did you feel about yourself? You know the answer: you might have felt good for your friend, but you felt bad for yourself, even for a moment. That is a natural reaction.

Your success in weight loss is likely to induce the same begrudging reaction in people around you. As I said before, it is normal. So, instead of getting worked up over this, be prepared to handle it.

One of the ways they might assuage their own guilt is by saying something along the lines of, "You have lost too much weight for your own good," or, "You look unhealthy," or even, "You look better with a little weight on you."

Take these comments with a pinch of salt. As long as your BMI is in the normal range, your weight loss is not unhealthy.

Long Trips

By this time, you should realize that weight loss and its maintenance require daily effort. Be aware that it may be difficult to maintain this tempo when you are travelling. While short trips of a day or two may not impact your regimen too much, longer trips have the potential to derail any regular habit.

An extended trip out of town can affect your weight management in many ways. You may not get an opportunity to weigh yourself daily, you may be exposed to a lot of buffet meals, and you may not have enough time to reach your daily quota of physical activity. To make things worse, when you get back home, you may have gotten so much out of sync that you completely throw in the towel on weight loss. This can be a really tough spot to get out of. Since this situation has the potential to undermine your effort in multiple ways, you need multiple defense mechanisms to save yourself from falling into this trap.

The first obstacle that you will encounter during your trip will be the non-availability of your scale. Although you may find a machine at your destination, I don't recommend using it. Most scales have some variability. An unusually higher or lower weight reading may throw you off track. The best option is to avoid weighing yourself on the hotel machines altogether.

Instead, you'll have to rely on your pedometer to keep you on course during your trip. Make sure that you bring your pedometer and it's charger. It will be a lifeline for managing your weight. Also be sure to use the treadmill in the gym to make certain that you hit your daily step targets.

While eating out, try to avoid buffet meals and elect the à la cart option wherever such an option exists. Employ all the tricks of handling buffet meals that I have taught you in a previous section.

Once you get back home, the first thing to do is to weigh yourself and compare that number with your weight when you left home. This will ensure that you immediately detect the impact your trip has had on your weight. If you've lost weight, seeing the number on the scale will be reassuring. However, in my experience, long trips usually lead to a gain in weight. If this is the case, the number on the scale will give you the necessary kick to get back on track immediately. Also keep in mind that you might feel reluctant to resume physical activity after a long trip. The only way to counter this is to not allow yourself any slack once you return home. Weighing yourself upon your return will act as a trigger to get you back on track.

The Weekend Trap

I am a professional and my work keeps me busy during most of the week. Early on, I recognized that it was much easier for me to adhere to my weight loss regimen on workdays than it was on weekends. First, we tend to eat more on the weekend. When you are a work, the opportunities for snacking are limited. However, when you are at home, you get many more opportunities to indulge. Second, we tend to eat out more often in a family setting. Both eating out and eating in company are known to significantly increase caloric intake.

To add fuel to the fire, caloric expenditure also goes down during the weekend. Unless your job requires to be chained to your desk, most people manage to accumulate a certain amount of steps at work. All these steps are taken out of the equation when you are at home.

Thus you are hit by a double whammy of increased caloric intake and decreased caloric expenditure over the weekend.

This is not just conjecture. In a 2014 study that monitored weight fluctuation, Brian Wansink from Cornell University found that weight increases over the weekend and decreases during the week. In fact, the researchers labeled this fluctuation a normal phenomenon. Even more relevant was their observation that people who are successful at losing weight or at maintaining the weight loss are the ones who are able to compensate for the weekend weight gain during the week.

A multi-pronged attack requires a multi-pronged defense. Let me share with you how I save myself from the scourge of the weekend weight gain. First, in order to compensate for the reduced baseline activity level, I make sure that I take my walks as early as possible. My daily target is 10,000 steps per day, so I try to get as close as possible to that many steps before 12 PM. I do this by taking a long walk in the morning, or having a rather long session on the treadmill. This leaves me very few steps to catch up during the day

I am aware that I get many more opportunities to eat during the weekend and the food is also more calorie-dense than my normal diet. I usually try to load up on things that are voluminous and yet low in calories. If I delay eating until late in the morning, I end up bingeing during breakfast. So I have a mini-breakfast of cereal before my actual breakfast or lunch. I also try to combine breakfast and lunch, which makes up for at least some of the extra calories. If I do go to a restaurant, I prefer to go to one that is located in a big mall. This way I end up walking a lot more going to and from the restaurant.

I allow myself at least one "day off" during the week. Typically, this period starts on Saturday evening and runs until Sunday evening. During this time, I may eat in a more carefree manner than usual without beating myself up about it. But I don't eat too excessively because I know that any excesses of the weekend will show up prominently on Monday's scale. This serves as the strongest motivation to get back on track during the week, when it is easier to restrict calories and achieve my daily step count goals.

Diet Food

These days there are many types of snacks and pre-packaged foods that are marketed as "diet" foods. Don't be fooled by the advertising. Most of these products contain almost as many calories as regular, "non-diet" food. Usually they contain less oil or fat and are frequently baked or roasted instead of fried. But still, the basic composition and energy density of the product is almost the same. It is the number of calories contained in a serving of a particular snack that is of paramount importance.

Consumers mistakenly believe that fat causes fat. This is the mistake. It is the extra calories that cause weight gain, not just the oil content.

Exercise Injury

It is very easy to get injured during any form of exercise, even while doing something as seemingly harmless as walking. Sometimes an injury is unavoidable and is an accident in real terms. What I am talking about here are the avoidable injuries. On many occasions, when you start exercising and begin seeing the results, you can become overly enthusiastic. You may start stretching yourself beyond your capabilities, and this can lead to exhaustion and injury. A common example of such a situation is when you are walking. You find that it is quite easy to do, and you try to go up from walking a couple of miles a day straight to doing double or even triple the distance. Or, you start running only a few days into your walking routine. These are examples of being penny wise and pound foolish. Remember that you cannot lose all your weight in one day. This is a marathon, not a 100-meter dash. Also, any injury to your legs will set you back much farther than the extra mile or two that pushing yourself would have set you forward.

To avoid this, create a daily target for yourself and stick to it diligently. You should ramp up your exercise efforts gradually as your strength and stamina builds up. This will go a long way in minimizing your chances of injury.

CHAPTER SEVEN

Staying Motivated

"People often say that motivation doesn't last. Well, neither does bathing — that's why we recommend it daily."
—Zig Ziglar, author, salesman and motivational speaker

Motivation to lose excess weight will initiate you on the path of the weight loss habit. Once your actions become habitual, they require progressively lesser effort to be sustained.

However, over a period of time fatigue may set in, which can lead you astray. If and when that happens, you will need an extra boost of motivation to get back on track again.

This completes the circle: motivation, habits, motivation. The key here is that you should be aware of the possibility of going off track, so that you can fix your course early on. As in other spheres of life, the farther you stray, the more difficult it becomes to return.

Over the years I have learned motivational techniques that have helped me get back on track whenever I veer off course. Familiarize yourself with these techniques and use them whenever necessary. These techniques are especially useful during those days, weeks or months when you find yourself with a net gain in weight.

Create Accountability

Right from our childhood, we learned to do certain things out of fear of retribution or ridicule. Hardly any child does their homework or brushes their teeth because he or she wants to. They do it because they are made to by their parents or teachers. We might have resented it back then, but as we grew, we not only realized the importance of that enforced discipline, but also sometimes missed it. I for one, miss it many times.

This type of accountability can be a powerful motivating factor for accomplishing anything. Luckily, you can create it for yourself even now and use it for your own good.

When you are planning to lose weight, consider sharing your decision and your weight loss goals with some close friends and family members. Go ahead and shock them with your impossible targets. Tell them, "By [date] I am going to be lighter by [number] pounds."

With one simple action, you will have recruited these people as your accountability partners. Right away, from the moment you tell them about your plan, they will start looking at you expectantly. The strength of this expectant behavior can be a strong motivating force. Just make sure you choose people with whom you are comfortable and who are truly in your corner.

"Don't break the chain"

Jerry Seinfeld, the famous comedian, was once asked about the secret of his success. Seinfeld revealed his system, which he calls "Don't break the chain." He explained that his livelihood depended on creating new jokes. New and effective jokes were the only "commodity" he had to offer to his audience. In order to push himself to produce new content on a regular basis, he committed himself to writing at least one new joke every day, all 365 days of the year. He bought a large calendar and would use a thick red marker to put a cross over the day he wrote a joke and continued to do that over a period of time until there was a chain of red crosses on the calendar. The longer the chain went by unbroken, the more important and valuable it became to him to keep it that way. So every day he would push himself to write at least one joke, just to be able to put that next cross on the calendar. "Don't break the chain." The beauty of the system is that it is not always just the one joke he would write. That was the minimum level required to get a cross on the calendar. On some days it would be more than one joke. At the end of the year he would have written a minimum of 365 new jokes.

The feeling of not wanting a chain to break is present in most of us. It is akin to the tendency to burst bubble wrap. No one tells us to do it, but it's in front of us, it's hard to resist. Similarly, when we're on a winning streak, we want to keep extending it. The longer it gets, the more valuable it becomes to us and the more motivated we are to do the work required to prolong it. By the way, Seinfeld used this technique to amass a fortune in excess of 800 million dollars. Your target is much smaller.

When you record your weight on a sheet of paper that includes your weight record for the entire month, you will automatically notice the weight entries of the previous days. If you skip a day, the blank space should prompt you to start the chain again.

A similar same chain can be created with your daily step count on the pedometer. I've had a target of doing 10,000 steps a day for almost five years. When a week goes by when every day I have been able to achieve 10,000 steps, a mini chain forms. Then, the week turns into a month-long chain and so on. My longest unbroken streak extended to almost six months, and only ended because of a neck sprain that required me to lie still in bed for almost two weeks. Boy, was I disappointed with myself.

So once you've created an unbroken chain going, be it with your weight log or your daily step target, you will find that it becomes progressively more precious and important for you to keep it going. This will provide the necessary motivation to stay on track.

Before and After Photos

When I started looking for information on weight loss, one of the first things that I came across were the success stories of people who had managed to successfully shed weight. Type the words "before and after weight loss" in Google and you will see literally thousands of pictures of people in both their fat and thin forms. You must see this for yourself. There are thousands of people who literally became unrecognizable after losing weight. These pictures can serve as a great source of motivation.

You might consider going a step further and creating your own set of "before and after" pictures. While pictures of other people who have lost weight can motivate you initially, your own before photo will keep you motivated farther on in the process. Seeing the numbers go down on your scale is one thing, but when you see yourself literally melting down, the feeling is exhilarating.

This is one of the most powerful motivators that I know of.

Old Weight Logs

Occasionally, I leaf through my old weight logs. The pages upon pages of entries that I have created over the years show a gradual but definite trend of declining weight. When I see some particularly old weight readings, I find it hard to believe that I ever weighed that much. This is why it is so important to keep your old weight logs. It is an invigorating feeling to see how far you have come. It reinforces your belief in your own capabilities.

A spreadsheet on a computer screen cannot convey the essence of the progress you have made in the manner that a hand written log does. This as another reason for keeping a hand written weight log.

A word of caution though. Don't fall into the trap of obsessing about these logs. I recommend that you go through only sporadically.

Become a Weight Loss Expert!

Once you start losing weight, you will find that people around you notice this change very quickly. I was surprised myself when people took note of my weight loss after I had lost only a few pounds.

You will get effusive compliments from people when you go to social gatherings. Get used to it! They will come up to you and ask about how you achieved your weight loss. Do share your techniques with them. I have seen some successful weight droppers who are modest, coy and even evasive about it. I don't see any reason to do that.

On the contrary, I found that sharing my weight-loss tips with people who wanted to know about them helped me even

CHAPTER EIGHT

Bonus Tricks

While researching for this book, I came across some interesting strategies that can facilitate weight loss. Many of them are a little off beat, hence I did not include them in the main text, as they may not have universal appeal.

However, I did see a lot of merit in them and didn't want you to miss out on their potential benefits. Each habit has the capability to either increase your caloric expenditure significantly or help you reduce your caloric intake. Either way, each of these habits has the potential to give an extra boost to your weight loss.

Game For Gum

Have you ever noticed how a cow is always chewing on something? Well, that effort does not go to waste; it is estimated that cows burn almost 20% of their caloric intake through their constant chewing.

I suspect that it was this fact that inspired James Levine of the Mayo Clinic to study the effect of chewing gum on caloric expenditure in humans. He set up an experiment to measure this precisely, using a machine called an indirect calorimeter. It is enough for us to know that this machine is big enough to seat a person inside it and measures the exact number of calories expended by that individual.

Levine found that for every hour of chewing gum, a person burns an extra 11 calories. Before you make light of this finding, consider the fact that this is same number of calories you would burn if you were to stand for an hour rather than sit in a chair. How does the deal look now?

Extrapolating this data, Levine estimated that if a person were to chew gum during all his waking hours, it would lead to a fat burn of 11 pounds per year.

I am not asking you to take this leap, nor do I think it is feasible. But you might consider chewing gum while you are driving or walking. 11 calories per hour for doing something that does not require you to even move your arms or legs, is not a bad deal at all, especially when you are fighting for every calorie.

Think of it as the interest you earn on your checking account. It might be a very minuscule return, but you might have a nice bonus by the end of the year.

2005 Super Bowl

During the 2005 Super Bowl, 40 graduate students at the University of Illinois' Graduate School of Library and Information Science were invited to a party on campus. They had agreed to participate in a food-related study in which they would be asked some questions.

As they marched into the venue, excited for the upcoming game, they were led into a room where snacks had been laid out . Unbeknownst to them, the experiment started the moment they started serving themselves.

The students had been divided into two groups randomly. Each group was led into a separate room which contained assorted roasted nuts and a pretzel/chip variety mix. The difference in the two rooms was that while in the first, the snacks were served out of four-liter serving bowls, in the other room they were served out of two-liter bowls. That was the only difference. Everything else was kept the same, including the plates and serving spoons. The students happily scooped out big portions of snacks for themselves and settled in for the game. No refills for the snacks were given, so they took whatever they thought would be enough to last for them through the game. Their plates were weighed before they started eating. After the game ended, their plates were weighed again, to determine the amount of snacks they had actually eaten.

The outcome of the experiment, amazed everyone involved.

The students who took snacks from the small bowls, each served themselves an average of about 52 grams of the mix. The students who were served out of the large bowls, on the other hand, each served themselves 80 grams of the mix. When the number of calories consumed by each group was measured, it was found that each small bowl participant consumed 251 calories and each large bowl participant consumed 393 calories.

The simple act of serving snacks from larger bowls led the students to consume almost 50% more calories those who were served from smaller bowls.

This study holds a simple lesson. Check your serving bowls. If you think it's possible to use smaller versions, go for it. This small change can have a huge impact on your caloric intake.

Still or Sparkling?

On my first visit to France, I went down to the hotel coffee shop in the morning to eat breakfast.

The server there asked me, in his accented English, "Still or sparkling?" (You have to imagine the accent part!) At that time I had no clue as to what was he asking. I learned later on, that, "still" referred to regular water and "sparkling" meant carbonated water, or club soda. I tried sparkling water a couple of times during that trip. Frankly, it appeared quite a strange habit to me to drink club soda instead of regular water with you meals.

Is it possible that sparkling water plays a role in making France the thinnest country in Europe?

An interesting study by Narumi Nagai from the Kyoto University, Japan seems to support my speculation. Essentially, Nagai fed a group of female volunteers regular water on one day and sparkling water on another day. Then using some advanced equipment that can measure fullness after eating and drinking, she compared both scenarios. Both types of waters raised the level of fullness experienced by the volunteers. But guess, which of the two caused more fullness? The sparkling water.

Some people have concerns about the safety of drinking carbonated water regularly. There is some speculation that it may be harmful. Rest assured, researchers have tried to look for potential negative effects of drinking carbonated water, but have not found any evidence. The only adverse effect that I have come across is that it may increase symptoms of gastric reflux in people who already are suffering from it. Other than that, there is no evidence that club soda produces any ill effects.

Drinking club soda with meals is an acquired taste so it may take a while before it starts to become enjoyable. If you end up developing a liking for it, you may have found an easy way of reducing your caloric intake.

Bon appetit!

Consider Keeping a Dog

There is plenty of evidence that having a dog can help you in more ways than one. Dog owners, especially those who take them out for a walk, end up walking almost 150 more minutes per week that people who don't have dogs. Almost 60% of dog owners take out their dogs walk. If you're part of the other 40%, consider assuming the responsibility.

Walking at Work

You might not know it, but there are treadmills available now that have fully functional desks built into them, allowing a person to work at a desk while simultaneously walking on the treadmill. How cool is that?

They were invented for the purpose of increasing the physical activity of people who are stuck in sedentary jobs. In fact, the idea was so appealing to some (myself included), that researchers conducted some major studies on their application and benefits in promoting physical activity.

Jamie Burr from the University of Prince Edward Island in Canada reviewed data on the use of treadmill desks at work and found that they help reduce both weight and abdominal girth. The benefits were even greater in obese people.

If you work from home and can start using a treadmill desk, it would be a great way to hit your daily step targets.

If you have any doubts about any harmful effects these desks might cause, rest assured. They do not impair your ability to work in any manner and have been found to be very safe.

So, if you are one the early adopters among your peers, do consider giving the treadmill desk a shot.

Size Does Matter

Scientists have long suspected that the size of your plate may influence the amount of food that you eat. A possible explanation is that we use dishware as a gauge to determine the appropriate amount to eat. Thus, if you use a larger plate or bowl, you will unwittingly serve yourself more food.

The idea is straightforward, but the results of research in this area are somewhat inconclusive. Scientists have made many attempts to measure the effect of using smaller plates on the amount of food people eat. For this, they have conducted many experiments in both real life and laboratory situations. Despite their best attempts, the scientists have not been able to prove conclusively that eating off of smaller plates will reduce your energy intake.

I have a contrarian view of the situation. I like to think that they haven't found any evidence of the opposite situation either, that is, that eating off of smaller plates increases your caloric intake. Until such a time that there is irrefutable evidence in this matter, my advice for you is to opt to eat off smaller plates whenever possible, especially in buffet type situations. It may not make a huge impact, but I don't see any harm either.

Extending this logic further, try using smaller serving dishes, plates, serving spoons and table spoons. Ever noticed the size of dessert spoons? They are usually much smaller than regular table spoons, the reason being that restaurants want you to enjoy dessert a little longer. You can use the same trick for the bulk of your meal.

Final Word

I wanted to summarise the key takeaways from this book at the end. I thought what better way than to visualise a typical day in your life once you have acquired the weight loss habit. As we go through this day in reference to the various habits discussed before, we would be able to cover the essential message that I have tried to convey to you through this book.

Let us begin right from the time that you wake up in the morning. You get up from your bed and get yourself a cup of coffee (tea if you prefer that). You make it either black, or use a dash of milk, no sugar added. Having finished your beverage, you wear your gym clothes lying next to your bed and as you pick up your cellphone and earphones, you also pickup your pedometer kept next to the them and wear it. You walk to a park a couple of blocks from your home and proceed to the jogging track. As you do that you switch on the run tracking app on the phone. You start walking on the track, listening to the latest episode of your favourite podcast. You finish your walk of 4 kilometres almost as the podcast also finishes. You then head back to your home and proceed to take a shower. As you come out of the bathroom, you weigh yourself, before wearing your clothes. You then make an entry of the day's weight and fat percentage in the diary kept next to the weighing machine. As you do that, you have a quick glance upon the previous days' entries. You notice that the day's weight is a couple of points over the previous day's weight and the fat percentage is almost same as before. You make a small mental note of this and get on with your day. Having worn your clothes, that fit you very well now, you wear your pedometer on your wrist and move to the kitchen for breakfast. There you pour a small cup worth of muesli into a bowl, add a couple of almonds and walnuts to it and then pour a cup of skimmed milk over it. Meanwhile, you set a frying pan on the stove and as it gets heated you make a small omlette with a couple of egg whites and some vegetables. You make this by using a combination of a non-stick pan and a very tiny dash of oil. You eat the breakfast, enjoying it all the way. Then you proceed to your workplace.

There you get on with your work and at around 11 A.M. you have another cup of coffee, made as you did in the morning and also eat an apple that you brought along from home. There you have a quick look at your pedometer and notice that your step count has reached 6500 steps, your target for the day being 11,000 steps. Then around noon you take out your sandwich made with brown bread, cheese, lettuce, tomatos and roasted ham/cottage cheese. You eat it slowly and drink a bottle of water with it. As you have some time at hand, you go for a small walk around your office block, thereby accumulating an extra 1500 steps in 15 minutes.

You come back home at around 5'O clock in the evening. As you enter your home, you go straight to the kitchen. There you make a large bowl of butterfree popcorn for yourself and have a cup of tea with it. Around an hour or so later you move to the dinner table. There, you start with thin tomato soup. Subsequently, you eat a bowl of casserole made with grilled chicken/ tofu and a couple of bread rolls made of whole grains. There is a caesar salad made to go along with it. For drinks, you have sparkling water. You end the meal with some fresh cut fruit and a small piece of dark chocolate. Meanwhile your pedometer vibrates, to indicate that you hit your daily steps target.

As soon as you finish your dinner, you go straight to the bathroom and brush your teeth thoroughly, thereby signalling the end of the day as far as the weight loss habit goes.

Of course, this is an oversimplification of the whole thing. The idea was to incorporate as many ideas as I could in one sample day. In real life, of course you will encounter thousands of different scenarios in terms of both eating and exercising. Yet, the basis crux of handling the days shall remain the same. Weigh yourself in the morning and make sure that you hit your steps target for the day. Rest of the habits shall will adjust and form around these two keystone habits. As long as you follow these two habits, you shall be the master of your weight.

Notes

Notes